The Ultimate Guide to Adult Videos

Ultimate Guides from Cleis Press

The Ultimate Guide to Anal Sex for Men
by Bill Brent

The Ultimate Guide to Anal Sex for Women
by Tristan Taormino

The Ultimate Guide to Cunnilingus
by Violet Blue

The Ultimate Guide to Fellatio
by Violet Blue

The Ultimate Guide to Pregnancy for Lesbians
by Rachel Pepper

The Ultimate Guide to Sex and Disability
by Miriam Kaufman, MD, Cory Silverberg and Fran Odette

The Ultimate Guide to Strap-On Sex
by Karlyn Lotney

The Ultimate Guide to Adult Videos

How to Watch Adult Videos and
Make Your Sex Life Sizzle

VIOLET BLUE

CLEIS
PRESS

Published in the United States by Cleis Press Inc., P.O. Box 14684, San Francisco, California 94114.

Printed in the United States.
Cover design: Scott Idleman
Book design: Karen Quigg
Icons: Courtney Sexton
Cleis Press logo art: Juana Alicia
First Edition.
10 9 8 7 6 5 4 3 2 1

LIBRARY OF CONGRESS CATALOGING-IN-PUBLICATION DATA

Blue, Violet.
    The ultimate guide to adult videos : how to watch adult videos and make your sex life sizzle / Violet Blue.
        p. cm.
Includes bibliographical references and index.
    ISBN 1-57344-172-4 (trade paperback : alk. paper)
    1. Sex instruction. 2. Video tapes in sex instruction. 3. Erotic films—Catalogs. 4. Video recordings—Catalogs. I. Title.
    HQ31.B58 2003
    613.9'6'0208—dc22
                            2003014823

Acknowledgments

A writer is nothing without her editor—and with this thought, I want to thank Felice Newman with all my heart for the invaluable contribution you made to this very multifaceted, groundbreaking work. Although now we work in unscripted concert, you show me what the combination of friendship and a matched love of work can do. And Frédérique Delacoste—ah! Do I have a crush on you? Maybe. But I'm definitely crazy about your sharp eye and superlative taste in design, and I still live for our conspiratorial smiles. Don Weise, whose work I admire greatly: Thank you for the long conversations, the hilarity when silicone overdose was imminent at *AVN*, and your friendship.

Constance, thank you for being my friend. You are simply one of my best friends, ever. Annalisa, my sweet, thank you for your friendship and support.

A very special thanks goes to my closest friend in the writing racket, the one person I turn to when I need an editorial favor, Sopranos-style. Thomas Roche, I am honored to be your friend, and I cannot thank you enough for helping me whenever I needed it.

Thank you, Carol Queen. You are the resource for all my tough questions, my sounding board for ideas. You always see the most interesting view, and you have a mind like a steel trap. You are one of my heroes.

Family is what makes us who we are, what makes us strong, what nourishes our psyches with love and support. Thank you to everyone in Survival Research Laboratories for being my family, and more. Thank you, Mark Pauline, for everything, including the teasing, the love, the respect, and for always being there—you are the closest family member of all. And Amy, thank you for the warmth and friendship.

This book would not have been possible without the hospitality of San Francisco's adult stores, where I ventured to rent stacks of porn. It was fun to go into these "no (wo)man's land" zones and discover other women shopping, too. Special thanks to City Entertainment on Folsom Street for all the help. And an extra-special thanks to Into Video in the Upper Haight for the handpicked videos in its stellar adult section and its knowledgeable staff—that's the store where the dream for this book was born.

A big thank-you to everyone who responded to polls, postings, and emails and consented to my interviews.

I save the best for last, like dessert. Which is just what you are, Courtney—the sweet part of my life. Thank you for taking care of me in every way imaginable (and even in ways I'd never thought of) when I was in the "heart of darkness" with this book. I'm always working on something, and you're always there for me, with more love than I thought was possible. Thank you for the coffee kisses, the flowers, pulling splinters out of my fingers, escapades with "motor oil," and chasing me around the house with your baritone horn. Thank you for everything. *Uz jsme doma*, my love.

Contents

Key to Icons and Ratings

The videos reviewed in this book are the cream of the crop, selected for quality, noteworthy scenes and performances, diversity, and superior filmmaking. They are made by people who take their craft seriously, and populated by performers who love their jobs. They are smart, original and created for sexually adventurous—and sophisticated—viewers who like to see hot sex done well.

Use the icons below to help you decide if a particular film has what you're looking for—or what you're trying to avoid. You'll find these icons accompanying each film review in the book.

Woman penetrates man. In these films, a man is penetrated by a woman either wearing a strap-on harness and dildo or using a hand-held sex toy.

Natural cast. Most, but not necessarily all, of the female cast members have natural breasts.

Unsightly boob job. One or more actresses have obviously fake breasts. You may see visible scars, rippling under the skin, unrounded shapes, or "frozen" breasts.

Well-made film. Big budget, excellent lighting, professional editing and camerawork, and care in setting up and executing scenes. This film could be a major release in all aspects of style.

Real female orgasm. The physiological signs are unmistakable: ejaculation, contractions, facial and body flush, uncontrolled muscular spasms. An actress in this film has a real orgasm onscreen. Yelling "oh god oh god" over and over again doesn't count. No fakers!

Sexually dominant women. One (or more) of the women is in charge of the action and demands satisfaction. Often indicates a female dominance scene.

Violet's Top Choice. If I gave out awards for great porn, these films would be the winners. Smart script, innovative premise, great story, hot sex, all of everything good and sweaty.

Intense chemistry. The chemistry between partners is obvious and hot, hot, hot.

Extreme sex acts. Caution! Contains choking, face-slapping, gaping, spitting on genitals or in face or mouth, or use of force that is not in an S/M context.

Great for first time viewers. Good starting point for viewers new to porn. You may find intricate plots, little or no hard-core sex, higher production values.

Foreword: They Shoot Porn, Don't They?

Throughout history people have enjoyed looking at sexually explicit imagery. Whether it be erotic temple paintings and sculptures that predate our Western world, calendars and stag films ("smokers"), or today's sophisticated porn videos and DVD's multiple angles and zoom close-ups, visual stimulation has for centuries been a significant part of our collective sex drives. In our visually rich, image-saturated contemporary culture, erotic visual stimulation is as viable and important a sex toy as ever.

Today, adult videos are so omnipresent, so readily available for any adult woman or man, that you'll have no trouble finding videos to rent or buy. Major cities and small suburbs have adult stores where hundreds, or thousands, of titles are available. And in the larger cities, you're likely to find that a noticeable number of these stores are owned or staffed by women. More than

11,000 titles are released each year (around 1,000 titles a month) in the United States alone, with target markets of men, women, and heterosexual couples of every stripe. The Internet is saturated with porn, good, bad, and ugly, from free to expensive. Website message boards and discussion forums about adult videos and DVDs get hundreds of new messages a day from both female and male viewers, and some of the most popular ones are moderated by women. More and more "straight" couples are watching porn each year, and according to comparative *Adult Video News* magazine statistics, the figures for female viewers are climbing. Meanwhile, women-run sex toy and video boutiques across the land are making their daily bread and butter from sales and rentals to women, couples, and (lastly) male consumers.

In fact, according to *AVN*'s annual sales and rental charts (*AVN*, January 2003), in 2002 more than eight million adult videos and DVDs were rented and over $900 million in revenues was derived from video and DVD sales alone. It seems clear from the statistics that in America watching porn is a fairly ordinary practice. I've watched those figures climb and met many of the people spending that money—and ask myself why, if there are so many of them (well, of us), are porn viewers still considered deviants by some? Indeed, if millions of Americans make this an entertainment choice each year, I believe that they are voting with their wallets and that they consider porn to be an inherently democratic pastime open to everyone with a TV and a VCR or DVD player. That's why I'm bothered that the media in general continue to paint virtually everything about porn in bold, negative strokes. I've long been suspicious of those media outlets, both print and broadcast, that condemn porn viewers and performers for their lifestyle choices—yet draw a hungry reader- and viewership with "shocking" details about the porn industry itself. Whenever media cover the adult video industry or viewership, it seems to me they wind up looking guilty of the same exploitation of which they accuse the industry and porn consumers.

Who, after all, are all these women and men watching all that porn? Evidently, a whole lot of regular people spending a great deal of money to spice up their solo and partnered sex with a practice they consider fun, natural, and harmless. And in my experience working at the women-owned and -operated sex toy boutique Good Vibrations, these consumers are a far cry from cultural stereotypes that depict porn viewers as deviants. What I found most intriguing five years ago, when I started helping customers find their videos, was that no particular type of customer fit any of the stereotypes I expected, and that sales and rentals of adult videos to all kinds of people were about to take off. Grinning boyfriends held piles of videos as their girlfriends picked them out and stacked 'em up. Hip grandparents were calmly making the most of a weekend alone with a few choice rentals. Solo women unblushingly picked up videos on rainy weeknights. Twenty-something guys of indeterminate sexuality browsed and rented porn tapes right along with the lesbians, butch dykes, gayboys, and straight couples, stepping up to the counter and discussing adult videos with me with no embarrassment or shame as if we were chatting about the latest predictable-but-entertaining Hollywood film. *All* of them were excited and intrigued to hear my opinions, ideas, fun facts about the films they were renting and buying, and my personal recommendations—and I loved our encounters, too. I've been reviewing and marketing adult videos ever since.

This book, then, is a product of my first-hand (so to speak) experiences with the world of porn. It's not feminist or antifeminist, politically correct or either for or against the adult industry. Rather, I've designed the book to be an entertaining, informative, lively tool that tells you how to get off using explicit videos, as well as how and where to find the exact videos that will suit your sexual preferences. This is not to say that every adult video will always be easy to take. You will discover, as I have discovered as a video reviewer and in compiling this resource, that adult videos can arouse and offend with equal ease. Porn can show you breathtakingly hot sex that can practically make you orgasm without touching yourself. It can give you erotic inspiration that takes your sex life to a whole new level. In it you can see women having authentic orgasms, couples so in love and in lust that your VCR might melt, sexual tension in both women and men that simply cannot be faked. Watching a porn video with your lover can ignite hot sex, sizzling conversations, or simply laughter at the ridiculousness of it all. Conversely, another video can put you to sleep or bore you to tears with rushed and uninterested sex, while still another can make you uncomfortable, or angry, with its horrifying racist depictions, lame female and male stereotypes, or unsafe sex practices. But I firmly believe that, at the same time you're experiencing any of these reactions (or, confusingly, several different reactions at once), you'll learn more about yourself and your own sexual needs, your relationships and desires, and human sexuality at large than you can from any other source in the world.

I entered the world of adult videos long before I worked for an adult store, watching videos alone and with my lovers. When I made the career jump to sex educator, video reviewer, and staffer serving customers, I felt as though I was beginning to witness something profound—something that I wanted to explain.

Everyone I spoke with, then and now, seemed hungry to understand more about my reactions and thoughts. However, some people I meet still jokingly refer to my "tough job" or my lucky boyfriend, and they occasionally comment seriously on how boring watching videos must be. Some assume that I want to be in the business, working in front of the camera—the implicit question being, what could a woman possibly get from watching porn? The question instead is, what does *anyone* get out of watching porn? The answers lie within these pages. I know that people's jokes, comments, and assumptions about my job come partly from envy, partly from curiosity, but mostly from a misunderstanding of who the female porn viewer is. Because that's what I am, in addition to my other roles: a female porn consumer. Yet most people who know me, or find out about my job, want to talk to me about it immediately and mine me for insider information about good videos to watch, where to find them, and tips on how to watch them. No problem. I have a plethora of advice and a list of recommendations long enough to fill an entire book. I hope *The Ultimate Guide to Adult Videos* helps you along the way as you explore the world of onscreen sex and perhaps come to enjoy adult videos as much as I have—and still do.

Violet Blue
San Francisco
August 2003

A Sex Toy Like No Other

Watching porn with my boyfriend has changed our whole sexual relationship. Now I have a better idea of what he likes, and I can take our sex games much further.

My friend Heather is a happy mother of three and wife of a computer programmer friend of mine. I love our conversations when I can quiz her about her work as a midwife—and when the kids are out of sight she loves talking to me about my writing projects. When I told her I was working on a book about using porn to enhance one's sex life, she looked astounded. Thinking I'd shocked her, I worried I'd overstepped our friendship's boundaries, until she blurted out, "A whole book about watching porn?! It's easy! You just get the tape you want, put it in the VCR, fast forward to the good parts, and go. It's that simple!"

What amounts to a simple "plug and play" equation for some people looms a daunting, unknown world to others. It's important to remember that everyone has a first-time experience watching porn, and each of us brings a unique mix of feelings and expectations to the moment. We hear from our friends that porn is hot, disgusting, fun, boring—or even all these things. That they were aroused, upset, had the best sex afterward, were uplifted, disappointed, embarrassed, inspired, or a combination of many feelings. Each individual's entry into the world of watching explicit sex onscreen is different—no two experiences are ever the same. But we all share the excitement that inspires us to try any new sexual experience.

The Porn Virgin

The first time I watched an adult movie, I went on the recommendation of a female friend of mine who knew a lot about porn. She listened to my list of desires—good filming, great story line, and a dark edge—and recommended a film that totally disappointed me. Part of the problem was that her interpretation of what I described as a "dark edge" was a film full of "tough guy" characters—quite different from what I wanted to see, as I had wanted something more crime-noir. But the main reason I ejected the tape after one scene was that I expected a movie like the ones I was used to watching in theaters, not the cheaply filmed, poorly constructed video I ended up with. I expected a regular *movie*. And alas, the very Los Angeles–looking and –acting actors in the movie turned me off, because they weren't anything like me or the people I could even imagine having sex with.

Getting myself to the point that I could comfortably select a tape I'd really like and get off while watching it was a matter of coming to know the unfamiliar, exciting, and arousing world of porn—a process of trial and error that involved watching many, many videos, both good and bad. I came to view the process of trying out new videos as an ongoing sex experiment, one that my lovers were often more than happy to help out with. In my head I had an idea about the type of video and situations I most wanted to see depicted, and allowed for that to change as I learned more about adult videos—and, at the same time, learned more about what turned me on. Now that I understand what I like, and how to find it, porn has become a sex toy that is as reliable to me as my trusty vibrator.

For newcomer and experienced porn viewer alike, porn can be a stocking stuffed with both candy and hand grenades. In this chapter, I offer a lot of suggestions that will help you define your fantasies and what you do—and don't—want to see in porn. Be prepared to spend money renting or buying videos that don't work for you; it's the only way to find what does. Once you understand more about the adult film world, you can be more specific when making your purchases or rentals, and you'll strike the jackpot more often than not.

Porn Myths and Stereotypes

Much like old myths that masturbation will make you go blind or grow hair on your palms—myths once intended to scare people away from exploring what we now know is a healthy sexual practice—a few myths tell about people who watch porn:

People who watch porn are compulsive masturbators.

Masturbation is normal. Everyone masturbates, and people who watch porn have a range of masturbation practices, just like everyone else. We live in a culture that labels anyone who enjoys masturbation as "compulsive," despite the normalcy of this healthy human behavior.

People who watch adult videos are porn addicts who can't enjoy sex without onscreen stimulation.

It's quite true that some people can become habituated to certain stimuli (especially when they discover something that works well), such as a frequent erotic fantasy, a pet vibrator, or a favorite sexual position. When you find something that you really like (or that brings reliable enjoyment to sex), repeat use does not mean you are "addicted" to it—though if you'd like to change your masturbation habits or broaden your range, you can adopt certain practices. Masturbation is the key method for incorporating new sexual practices, and by arousing yourself with masturbation by familiar methods, you can try new sexual behaviors while in your most familiar state of heightened arousal. Turn yourself on and try something new.

People who watch porn are child molesters.
Or: Watching porn turns people into rapists and child molesters.

People who molest children are interested in children, not adult porn. Those interested in sexualizing underage kids will be much more interested in watching movies that feature young children than masturbating to explicit, healthy adult sex onscreen. Adult videos are voluntary arousal tools, like sexual fantasy (the imagination), erotic books, and sex toys, to name a few. They lack the power to "make" anyone do anything they do not already want to do.

Only people who can't have a "real" relationship watch porn.

This is one of the most hurtful myths, designed to shame people into sexual isolation. Retail statistics chart the skyrocketing sales and rentals of porn to couples, showing that couples as well as unpartnered individuals are using porn to enhance their relationships or to find release in between relationships. Some choose solitary pleasure, and porn provides a great release from sexual tension. Besides, taking time out to masturbate when you're in a relationship isn't cheating—it's taking care of yourself.

When you watch porn, you support a racist/sexist industry.

I partially agree on this one. Sexist stereotypes in porn? They're like wheat in Kansas. Racist stereotypes in porn? You bet. These issues have been huge struggles and pivotal turning points for many performers and directors, and thankfully, these directors and performers have turned these stereotypes on their heads, striking back and making their own, hot, smart, porn—porn that even erotically comments on these stereotypes. To escape the clichés, look for videos made by women, people of color, and independent production houses.

Porn makes viewers want more extreme sex or sexual material.

That's like saying if someone tries hot sauce, they'll never be happy until they set their tongues on fire. Perhaps for some—but really, is Edward

Penishands a gateway drug? Watching adult videos does not give you some unquenchable thirst to find something crazier, harder, more extreme—you already have this urge before you turn on the TV. It's true that when you grow comfortable with porn you will crave variation—but within the bounds of what's sexually comfortable for you.

Who Watches Porn

Take a stroll to your local library, grocery store, movie theater, or mall, and you'll have made contact with lots of people who watch porn. Like the pod people in *Invasion of the Body Snatchers,* they can't be recognized just by looking at them—except maybe they've got a little more spring in their step. Adult movie viewing is still as taboo a subject as masturbation in our culture, but most people have caught a glimpse of porn, and an awful lot watch it regularly. The stereotype of the furtive man in the raincoat has faded like a B-movie special effect into our past; today women, men, and couples of all orientations and of all walks of life participate in one of our favorite extracurricular activities: watching adult films.

Millions of average people a year in the United States rent, purchase, and enjoy porn. Porn is not just watched by single men but by women, men, and couples—with a diverse range of age, physical ability, sexual orientations, and backgrounds. Although men have typically been (and still are) the largest consumers of porn, women and heterosexual couples are quickly adding their numbers to viewership statistics. Women-owned sex toy businesses that cater to female customers added explicit films to their stock only about fifteen years ago, and when they did they saw their businesses grow exponentially. Many of these women-owned sex shops see their porn sections as a reliably increasing area of revenue, and for these shops, single men are the shopping minority.

According to annual rental charts published in the industry journal *Adult Video News,* stores in the United States reported over 800 million rentals of adult tapes for 2002 (*AVN,* January 2003). While a 1997 study by the Society for the Scientific Study of Sexuality concluded that most explicit books, magazines, and videos were marketed to heterosexual men, the researchers noted that in previous years an increasing amount of material had been produced by and for heterosexual women.

The adult business has responded to the change in viewership. In the 1970s and 1980s, pretty much the whole genre was being produced with men in mind, despite a number of notable exceptions. *Deep Throat* caused a stir of epic proportions showcasing an outrageous sex act, and even celebrities flocked to seedy movie houses to see it. At the same time, *Behind the Green Door* showed to an enthusiastic audience at the 1972 Cannes Film Festival. As a result, women and heterosexual couples became visibly active consumers. Through the 1990s women-owned sex shops became steady sellers of porn, and the industry sat up and took notice. Not only were these businesses proving profitable, but other adult retailers were starting to realize that women were statistically increasing their market presence through purchasing power—and lots of couples were watching porn, too. The industry responded by producing movies that they thought women too might want to watch.

Today women are watching porn in increasing numbers, and to my mind it's a happy sign of a much-needed change in women's sexual roles. In our culture, women simply aren't exposed to as much explicit sexual imagery as men are, but this is all changing. One of the major obstacles that we women face in determining our own healthy vehicles for sexuality is the widely held notion that women don't respond to sexual imagery as men do—a notion that is absolutely untrue. In her 1994 study, Dr. Ellen Laan of the University of Amsterdam proved that women do in fact respond physiologically to sexual images, even when they said that the porn they watched was boring or unarousing. When seeing sex onscreen (whether from male or female directors), the women in the study responded, their genitals becoming congested with blood—a hallmark of the sexual response.

Why Watch Porn?

In the quest to self-define our own healthy sexualities, let's pull back the curtain on all these average folks who watch porn. What are all these people using these dirty movies for? Why would anyone watch porn—and what can you get from it? The men and women who like porn have their own range of motivations. Most just want to get off seeing people have sex—it's that simple. Quite a few enjoy the notion that it's dirty to see anyone, especially women, being aggressive and explicit sexually, and the taboo titillates them. Explicit sex onscreen seems to be a powerful aphrodisiac for lots of people—and maybe it will be for you, too. It could be that you want to try out porn as a sex toy, the same way you might buy a new vibrator or play with a different brand of condom. Or the idea of doing something forbidden, naughty, or "dirty" might be your sexual flavor of the month. Maybe the idea of watching two people get it on is on your top ten list of sexual fantasies. Whatever your attitude, porn is the safest way to watch, period. There are many reasons to watch adult videos, and you may find one, or several, of your motivations here.

To Get Off

The simplest, most basic reason to watch porn, of course, is "to get off." Many people use adult videos just as another person would use a vibrator—like a sex toy. Switch it on, it gets you aroused and pushes you over the top, then switch it off and put it away. You can masturbate to porn any way you like, anytime. It can be a fantastic sex toy that keeps you sexually healthy, in touch with your own arousal and orgasms, and visually in touch with what sex looks (and sounds) like. Porn can get you revved up before you go out, or it can be part of a hot date you have with yourself. Explicit visual stimulation has such a powerful arousal trigger—especially sex acts, scenes, or fantasy scenarios that fulfill a particular fantasy—that most people (men *and* women) can use it reliably to bring themselves to orgasm.

Curiosity

One big reason you might be interested in watching an adult film is to find out what the big deal is. Curiosity is a force to reckon with. Porn is everywhere: in the media, on TV specials, the topic of blockbuster movies. Porn stars are in glossy magazines, and you may have a friend or lover who has talked about watching adult videos—or bragged about dating a porn star. None of these things actually shows you any porn, or gives you an idea of what the movies, or their effects on you, are really like. Perhaps it's time to end the mystery.

To Get a Different Kind of Education

In California, around 1980, most of us who were kids in fourth grade were treated to a grand total of one hour of sex education. This consisted of the boys and girls being separated and shown animated films about reproductive anatomy, puberty's physiological changes, and the cycle of birth. It was great to learn where babies came from, I thought, but in terms of the whole of human sexuality and what we were going to discover as we became adults, these films didn't seem related to sex at all. No one told us about pleasure, or what sex—or even actual, nonillustrated genitals—looked like. Many children didn't even watch sexual education films in school.

Porn can make up for this deficiency many of us share, and become part of your own personal erotic education. You might watch it to learn new techniques or moves, or to see how the pros do it. Although the people in porn usually don't look like "average" people—they're relatively skinny, augmented, made-up, and shaved or waxed—when they get down and dirty they show us what it looks like when people have sex. It's a wholly different type of sex education, and an essential one at that. Unless you make love in front of a mirror or look at your (and your partner's) genitals up close, you may never have an accurate idea of what realistic genital topography is or what people actually look like when they are being sexually stimulated. For people who have concerns about how their genitals look, or feel discomfort with how their bodies look, it's an eye-opener to see someone else's genitals eroticized—especially if they look like your own. My sexual education grew by leaps and bounds as I watched porn, simply because I saw a variety of types of anatomy, and I truly got an education when I saw my first up-close female ejaculation, pulsing urethra and all. While porn isn't great for learning about accurate sex techniques (since the editing means that the whole of sexual activity isn't necessarily shown), it can—sometimes inadvertently—be an amazing learning tool in this respect.

A Sex Toy for Two

Glossy men's magazines like *Maxim* run plenty of articles that tell guys how to convince their women to watch porn with them. So what's the allure for couples to try it? Easy—it's another sex toy that couples can share. The first time you try it, watching an explicit film is an experiment; you'll either think it's lame and turn it off, hopefully laughing, or you might feel a twinge of arousal…maybe more. And it can be fun for you both to watch hot sex, and both be turned on at the same time. Porn is a versatile toy, too, because you can take turns watching, use your hands, imitate the people onscreen, or use the imagery to spark desire and ignore the film altogether. How you use it together is up to you.

Couples who want to add a little spice to their sex lives can find porn to be a fun way to turn up the heat. Conversely, they may watch a few films, find them anticlimactic (pardon the expression), and have hotter sex because they know they can do it better than the porn stars—and because porn *can* lack heat and chemistry between couples, it's likely true. But check your expectations: Being a sex toy, porn only enhances what you've already got; it cannot replace or "fix" anything.

New couples can add porn to an already-sizzling sex life to push their new sexuality to higher levels, or into new territory. Established couples, especially those with children or other time constraints, might enjoy having a very special adult "treat" that they can enjoy in their private time together. Those who find they like this versatile sex toy can add regular viewing to their sexual repertoire, perhaps mixed in with other variations like fantasy play and sex toys. Read all about how to watch porn together, and introduce your lover to porn, in Chapter 2, "How to Watch Porn."

Find New Fantasies

To tell the truth, by and large lots of porn is pretty unimaginative. It falls into basic formulas, and the scene endings are, well, predictable. But adult film is one of the only industries in the world actively, endlessly exploring and enacting human sexual fantasies, always on the lookout for new scenarios, for new and exotic locations, for new ideas to depict on film, and even for new positions and sex acts to show the viewer. This makes it a unique place to look for new material for your own fantasy life, as it can give you new ideas of things to try with a lover or a date. Often the scenarios might seem mundane, but you'll likely be surprised by the power of your libido when you become aroused seeing something from a fresh angle, or see a position you'd like to try, or even realize that you want to experiment with a new type of sex act, such as oral sex or S/M.

It's Just Something Different

Tired of the same old thing when you masturbate? You're not alone—the popularity of sex toys in general underscores the fact that most people enjoy variety in their masturbation. Porn is just another way of stirring the pot.

Watching Something You'd Never Try Yourself

Sexual fantasies that you use for masturbation often don't have a lot of grounding in reality, or if they do, they're likely unrealistic in a big way—that's why they're *fantasies*. And that's okay; it's perfectly acceptable to fantasize about things you'd never actually try, or even ask someone else to do. Sometimes you might find that these fantasies are beyond what you'd deem permissible for you to try in real life, and they might even seem disturbing. But know this: Just because you fantasize about something doesn't mean you want it to come true. Fantasies of all stripes, from the benign to the extreme, can be found in porn, and this makes adult film an especially suitable arena to see something you'd never try yourself, but might enjoy masturbating to. This can range from fantasizing about same-sex erotic activities to getting off watching something you find potentially offensive—like facial come shots or scenarios involving a hint (or a lot) of force. If it offends or really bothers you, then don't do it—but if you realize that you're simply watching consenting adults who seem to be enjoying themselves, and that watching them at play doesn't change your identity in any way, you might feel free to use your forbidden fantasies to their full erotic potential.

To Get What You Can't Find at Home

Porn can be a great way to introduce a new erotic activity, such as oral or anal play, into your sex life. What if, over time, you realize that you'd like to try a new sexual activity with your lover, such as oral sex, and you ask her or him to try it, and your partner claims not to be interested? Well, you can drop the subject, never breach it again, and mourn the loss of fulfilling a potential fantasy with your lover—though you may wind up frustrated and resentful over time. I don't recommend this route. You could also cheat on your partner, but that's almost always disappointing and ends badly. You could badger your partner, but that's no solution, either. You have a better choice: Address your dilemma with little or no damage to your relationship, *and* find a satisfying way to enjoy your fantasy—by watching other people "do it" in a hot adult film.

So if your lover absolutely hates the idea of wearing a strap-on and penetrating you with a commanding attitude and forceful demeanor, you can rent or buy a film like *Bend Over Boyfriend* and watch other real-life loving couples engage in anal sex—and you can get off on a vicarious thrill. You can even tell your lover that this is the solution you'd like to seek, though do so gently, and reassure your partner that this isn't a substitute for her or him—simply a way for you to have your fantasy realized within your relationship. If your partner seems open to the idea, you can invite her or him to watch with you. Read more about trying new things with a reluctant partner in Chapter 2, "How to Watch Porn."

When your sweetie comes around to wanting to watch porn with you, you can use the video you choose as a vehicle for bringing up a sex act you're interested in, one that might seem otherwise out of place to talk about in any other context. You can be watching a scene that contains something you find sexually interesting, like a threesome, and see how your partner feels about it—sort of test the waters before you actually express your desires about making it come true. You can comment on the sex act, ask your partner what he or she thinks of it, and chances are good that either you'll know right away that your partner isn't interested, or you'll have the perfect opportunity to start talking about it as a fantasy for you both to share.

Visual Arousal

When we think about desire, erotic attraction, and arousal, we give all the credit to the functions of the higher brain—the thinking functions. We believe in our free will, our skills in making decisions to guide the more mysterious, more animalistic urges around sex. It's long been a hallmark of human nature that our sexuality is under volition; as rational people we have no doubt that healthy sexuality requires self-control. Not a scrap of our sexual fantasies and desires (or so we think) is left completely on automatic pilot, just as even when we drive a car we consciously stay on the road. At least until we see someone we're attracted to—and suddenly desire turns us right into monkeys, and we start acting like them.

Meaningful sexual motivation, it turns out, has little to do with physiological arousal. In fact, we get turned on by what we see, or by imagining or visualizing a sexual fantasy. Such visual creatures are we that our entire world is made up of images and feelings, together with the emotions and desires they trigger. At the same time, relationships are the bread and butter of who we are, intimate relationships a delicious main course for our psyches—yet graphic erotic imagery sends a direct current buzzing from our brains to our groins. Images turn us on, and they can get us off. That is, if we use them properly.

Relationships and arousal from pornography may come from two different places, yet they aren't mutually exclusive. In our ideal relationships, the conscious act of desire and genital performance are not things we want separated; instead we want the two working in tandem, like a perfect set of doubles in tennis. But porn is so immediate, so visceral, that it disrupts our rationality. We can't help but look at it, nor can many of us resist getting aroused by it. And because we want our throbbing erections and wet pussies to play nice with our relationships, the lack of control makes us feel like suddenly we're driving a car with no brakes. It's as if what's safe is always at odds with what is sexy. It doesn't have to be, but the act of bringing the two ideas together is a conscious one. It takes examining what porn really is, and how to use it.

Some people feel as intimidated by porn as they do by sex toys—though that's all porn is: a sex toy in a thousand different guises. It's an arousal tool to use with a partner, or alone. Watching adult videos is still considered by most people to be something "dirty." But watching porn in most cases is simply a means to an end: the watcher's orgasm. End of story, and sleep tight. Watching erotic videos can spice up a night at home with a lover, or be a solo masturbator's quick and reliable way to relieve sexual tension. People watch porn to get off on visual stimulation, because watching sex, sexy images, or fantasy scenarios makes us hot. And nothing gets to the point better than porn.

Your Fantasies in Living Color

Porn takes sexual fantasies (and fantasy sex acts) out of the realm of imag-ination and puts them up on the big screen, or the wide-screen TV, for all to see. Sexual fantasy is everyone's own private, personal sex toy. A good fantasy played out in your head can take you to dizzying heights of arousal, enhance an intensely private moment of masturbation, or illu-minate an experience with a partner. Someone can have a scenario progressing in their head when receiving oral sex, act out their impulses with a companion, or tell their fantasies to a lover on the phone. But before we turn our fantasies into the unforgettable encounters we wish them to be, or prepare to see them onscreen, we first have to define what they are.

Sexual fantasy is the cornerstone of our individual sexual expression. An erotic fantasy is any thought, idea, image, or scenario that interests you sexually. It doesn't necessarily have to turn you on, or by contrast it can be the one thing that gets your blood boiling. And if you think you don't fantasize, think again. Fantasies can emerge from your erotic imagination in countless different forms, from fragmented to detailed. We may see famous people who are attractive and imagine that our lives overlap. We can revisit memories of times we have enjoyed, using them to make us feel good in the present. Often, we envision scenarios that have never happened—and some that aren't even possible.

Sometimes we tell others what we have actually done, fantasized about, or want to do, making a fantasy for them—or us—come true. Whatever shape your fantasies take, exploring them can open doors to understanding your arousal, while allowing you to tap into new channels of erotic expression that work for you.

Some people don't care to explore their fantasies. Many others are more willing. Because those fantasies arise in our imagination, and there-fore are connected with our subconscious, they can be startling, unpredictable, and sometimes even shocking. When we become aroused it's easy to surrender ourselves to whatever movie we're running in our heads, and push it in the direction that gets us closer to orgasm—but sometimes, afterward, we realize that what got us off went beyond what we deem acceptable in our daily lives. It's easy to feel guilty after a fan-tasy has gone to a place or an act we find unpleasant or offensive. Admitting this guilt can make us feel shame about sex, our desires, even who we are. Especially if the fantasy was powerful and included some-thing that in real life we would never do, like degrade ourselves or betray a loved one. When fantasies move toward the arenas of everyday life (as they are bound to do), they can manifest in ways that make us uncom-fortable.

Sometimes it's not the content of the fantasies that can trigger guilt, but rather the time or place that they occur. Fantasies can happen at inconvenient times, such as at work or on the bus, creating a sexually charged situation in our heads while the world goes on around us. This may feel inappropriate or "dirty." Or they can happen during sex with a partner: Your partner is fully present, yet unaware that you are imagining things, even acts with other people, to get yourself off. You might mastur-bate to your memory of a scene in an adult movie you saw without your partner—or you might witness your secret fantasy while your sweetie is sitting right next to you. The illusion is created that somehow we've betrayed them. It's important to understand the role of sexual fantasy in sex before beating yourself up about what, how, with whom, or when you fantasize.

We all know that fantasy is not reality. But when we masturbate and imagine troubling things, people, or situations, our human curiosity kicks in and we ask ourselves whether these things are what we really want. For some people this is a horrifying thought. It's important to keep in mind that fantasies don't necessarily bear any relationship to reality. The realm of fantasy is the sanctuary in your mind where you are free to enjoy things that you would never do in real life. And fantasy is not only where we can court the forbidden, it is also a powerful sex toy that can be used to arouse, heighten pleasure, and achieve climax.

Common Fantasy Themes

Think about your fantasies for a moment, whether they are vivid, vague, seemingly mundane, or a little scary. Don't try to look deeply into their meanings, just pick out their main themes. What you're doing is isolating what makes them a peak erotic experience for you. Keep your mind open, and don't pass judgment on yourself—this isn't about "good" and "bad," it's about understanding what turns you on. Note what stands out, and weigh the important differences between what is possible in fantasy and what is possible in reality. The list below can also help you make the right selections when looking for a porn film that will get you off. Here are some themes:

- Firsts (first time with a sexual act such as penetration, oral sex, or anal sex)
- Loss of control (someone has sexual power over you, "makes" you do things)
- Having control (exerting sexual power, having people "service" you)
- Taboo (with a forbidden person like clergy or family, an animal, same gender, significant age differences, inappropriate urges or timing, rape, nonconsent)

- Multiple partners (a gang bang—one person with four or more partners; sex with the football team; threesome; sex party; orgy)
- Casual or anonymous partners (strangers, the waitress, the UPS guy)
- Your current or past partner (a memory of a real-life event; imagining a peak experience you hope to do together; imagining your partner behaving differently than usual, such as being dominant or submissive)
- Public spaces (the last row in the movie theater, a shaded spot in the park, a department store dressing room, over your desk at work)
- Being "used" (a slave, a fuck toy, getting passed around)
- Role play (you or your partner as an icon: a cop, schoolgirl, hooker, doctor, teacher, human pony, dog owner)
- Gender play (seeing women as men, men as women, or people who are both—that is, transsexuals)
- Romance (dreamy settings: being seduced by a rock star or actor, making love tenderly to the girl at the office, being rescued by a hot and horny fireman, saving your sexy fantasy lover from danger)
- Objectification/fetish (breasts, butts, dicks, mouths, panties, shoes)
- Voyeurism (watching people have sex through the bushes or outside their house, secretly seeing a man or woman undress or masturbate, watching people have sex on TV, seeing other people—such as a single woman—watch sex acts)

Now you're getting an idea of your main fantasy components. Think about what your favorite themes are, or try on new ideas that appeal to you. Feel comfortable with tapping into what these fantasies trigger when you want to become aroused. Remember that if you fantasize about something shocking, like being forced to perform sex, it doesn't mean that you want it to happen or that you are a bad person. But by identifying it in the realm of your fantasies, you can find a safe space where imagination fuels desire. By learning how to turn yourself on with fantasy, you can do extraordinary things, like make yourself really aroused and teach yourself a new masturbation technique. Or you can fantasize while your partner goes down on you, and learn to orgasm with the combination of their stimulation plus your fantasy. If you have a partner, and have established trust and sexual communication, you can share your fantasies—you can even make some of them come true. And if you're shopping for the right adult movie, with some sizzling fantasies on your mental checklist you'll have a better idea of what you want to avoid—or what you really, *really* want!

CHAPTER

2

How to Watch Porn

I got so turned on that I had to leave the room, and I masturbated in the bathroom. It was the dirtiest thing I'd ever done, running off to finger myself. I didn't know that women—that I—could have an instant "erection!"

Watching porn is inherently sexy. Enjoying the visual stimulation it provides is a natural sexual act, and adding it to your sex life can open up a whole new avenue of sexual expression. Individuals, couples, and even groups of friends watch porn together for a variety of reasons, employing a wide range of activities and practices, with myriad results. How you incorporate porn into your sex life is entirely up to you.

Watching porn on your own can be terrific for first-timers or a reliable source of ongoing erotic entertainment for porn enthusiasts. What's better, one-on-one experiences with porn can help us reclaim elements of our sexuality (such as fantasy and mastur-bation) that are missing from our cultural definitions of healthy sexual expression. Private access to free, uninhibited sexual enjoyment is possible with the visual stimulation that porn provides, and this freedom is our sexual birthright. Solo viewers can let go and be themselves, emotionally, physically, and mentally—for learning how to watch porn for personal enjoyment is liberating, empowers us, and builds personal sexual autonomy.

Sharing adult videos with a lover can take an important, central part of your relationship—shared sexual intimacy—to deeper levels of sexual connection. Watching together provides assurance about the naturalness of your sexual expression, and may strike (or fan into flame) the erotic spark. Many couples report having incendiary sex when they watch porn. Some get turned on together while watching other couples get it on. Others like to act out what they see onscreen. Couples use porn together to break the sexual ice; once the film starts they may find they can't keep their hands off each other. The film may inspire a conversation about something they'd like to try, such as anal sex or role-playing. Some will watch a film all the way through, then go to bed and do what they usu-ally do—only hotter. Telling my lover I have to watch a film for "research" purposes—and that I need a research assistant—works like a charm.

The context for your first adult video may not intentionally be a sex-ual one, solo or otherwise. You might watch your first porn film when your best friend drags you to a bachelorette party, or when a pal suggests something "wild," like renting a dirty movie. If you decide you're okay with going along for the ride, know that you're doing just that—it's likely that your friend or friends were too nervous to watch porn on their own, and wanted to have you there to make it feel safer. It can be a lot of fun to watch porn with friends, and with the right crowd you might wind up laughing your head off. Prepare yourself by knowing that there's a chance you might see something that will arouse you or offend you, and realiz-ing that, you'll be better able to disengage from seeing explicitly sexual material with people you don't feel sexual about. However, if you'd like to consider adding porn to your erotic repertoire, I recommend that you watch your first adult film alone.

Solo Viewing

Since most porn is viewed alone, you'll be joining the millions of women and men who regularly take time out for themselves for solo pleasure with their erotic video of choice. Solo porn viewers know what they like, enjoy trying new things, are confident in making their own sexual choices, and like to treat themselves to masturbation on their own time and on their own terms. This reality is light years away from the false stereotype of porn viewers as raincoat-clad, drooling, compulsive masturbators. Whether done by a gal enjoying time with her roommates gone, the mom with a quiet evening to spare, a man whose girlfriend is out of town for the weekend, or the guys who visit peep-show video booths on their lunch hour, watching porn ignites routine masturbation with a visceral erotic spark.

When you watch your first adult video alone, you'll be doing it without anyone else around to make you feel self-conscious, nervous, or worried about how you are feeling or reacting to what you see onscreen. That includes your lover, your best pal, the hottie you want to seduce, and anyone who might interrupt you with an uncomfortable surprise. Make sure your housemates are really not coming home, your kids are away, your sweetie is at work—check off all important items on your mental list so that you'll have total solitude and privacy.

When you get those videotapes in your hot little hands and are all ready to spend some time alone with the VCR or DVD player, make sure you have everything you need and will be undisturbed. If you can, eliminate possible distractions. Nothing is worse than taking your erotic temperature by watching your first adult film, getting turned on, and experimenting—and then having the phone ring, bringing your arousal crashing down to earth. Unplug or turn off your phone, and don't try to multitask with any chores. Focus on checking out the video. You may or may not like it or even get turned on, but you'll want to be able to assess for yourself how you feel. If you're worried about privacy and sound, make a mental list of what will make you feel safe; close your doors and windows, and keep the volume at a comfortably low level.

Now set the scene for your adult video viewing adventure. Wear loose clothing, or clothes that you can easily reach into if you find yourself in the mood and wanting to play along with the folks onscreen. Pajamas or a robe work well. Make a place to view the screen that's comfy to sit or lie back in, or cuddle up with a blanket. You may be planning on masturbating, or could wind up masturbating unplanned, so have a towel handy. Lube is nice, and a favorite vibrator is a highly recommended companion to the remote control. You might not use the extra items if the movie doesn't meet your criteria—but it's nice to have the gear when you want it.

You can watch a movie on the sly, when no one is around, or you can also make it a hot date with yourself. Treat yourself to a luxurious shower or bath to relax, a really sensuous one if you like. Have something special to nibble on or sip, and play some music that is especially relaxing or sexy for you as you prepare. Before you start the tape, take a minute to touch yourself erotically, teasing and arousing yourself. You can even get yourself in the mood by masturbating a little before the movie starts.

Three Cheers for Masturbation

I'm enthusiastic about masturbation. It's is the cornerstone of our sexuality—the arena in which we build our fantasies and learn how we like to be touched. Masturbation offers a source of release on many levels. Unfortunately, our culture has a restrictive view of it and tends to shroud masturbation in a cloak of shame or failure—but that is changing. Still, some people might see masturbating to porn as a negative thing: a self-defeating substitute for partnered sex, a secret shame, an admission of guilt. These ideas are damaging, and if you are coping with these feelings when you want to masturbate while watching erotic imagery, consider what effect these self-deprecating thoughts may have on your emotions today and your emotional state in the future.

Masturbation is nature's way of letting us release tension and boost self-esteem, while it teaches us sexual self-reliance. It's a positive, life-affirming practice that can help all of us cope with depression, doubt,

Tips for Solo Viewing

LEARN YOUR OWN SEXUAL anatomy before turning on the TV. Read a good sex guide that covers anatomy, sit down naked in front of a mirror, or allow your hands to explore your genitals.

Set aside some time for yourself when you have no obligations and some privacy. Treat yourself to something nice and sensual first, like a relaxing shower or bath, a new lubricant, or comfy clothes and a snuggly blanket.

Set yourself up with things you won't want to interrupt the action to retrieve, such as the remote, a towel, lube, a vibrator, a dildo (or any other sex toy), something to drink, and an emergency cover like a blanket.

Start the video, but pay more attention to yourself first. Using lubricant, caress your genitals with your hands, spending time to linger in the spots that feel good. Familiarize yourself with the different skin textures and colors, and take note of your favorite spots.

Tease yourself. When something feels really good—as in "imminent-orgasm!" good—back off and touch yourself somewhere else, such as your nipples. This prolongs your pleasure and can make your orgasm really intense.

Try masturbating in different posi-tions. You can sit in a chair, lie on your belly or back, or experiment with legs open or closed.

If you'd like to learn a different technique for masturbation or orgasm, get yourself aroused—very aroused—watching a scene that gets you hot while using your regular masturbation technique. Slowly begin to introduce the new behavior, such as trying anal penetration. You can also use this arousal to try things that may be ordinarily challenging, like deep throating a dildo. You can also experiment with prolonging orgasm. It may not catch on the first few times, but it will as you continue to incorporate it into your pleasure cycle.

Indulge yourself! Let your fantasies run wild. Become anyone, including the people onscreen. Orgasm as many times as you can—or come quickly, and hard. Be as nasty or as sweet as you like, and relish spending some truly decadent time giving yourself much-earned plea-sure. Forget about the rest of the day; this time is for you. You're taking time out to take care of yourself and your body, and to make yourself feel good—something we never do enough. You deserve it!

anxiety, and grief. Plus, it stimulates blood flow to our genitals, keeping them healthy. Many people find masturbation very healing, in or out of relationships. Everyone can use masturbation to consciously learn orgasm and orgasmic control, and it is the primary means of teaching yourself new ways to get off. It's the golden key to learning how to reach orgasm, period! You can teach yourself to come with penetration and with a partner, or you can train your body and mind to achieve orgasms any way you desire. Masturbation feels great, it's good for you, it can make partnered sex absolutely delightful, and it can keep you grounded.

There's a stereotype that people who get off to porn only watch it by themselves, or that if someone watches porn he or she must not be in a relationship. This idea is sometimes used in a derogatory way, as if to say that single people only watch porn because they're desperate for a relationship, or incapable of having one. This may be true for some people, but whether you're in need of a quick release or just want to get off alone, singles have the same variety of reasons for watching porn as do couples. In fact, single people have a lot to gain. Porn is a fine tool for sexual pleasure when you're alone. No one likes to feel sexually frustrated, and using explicit images to masturbate to is a great way to find release. Some people are simply more comfortable with solo sex and pornography than they are being with a partner, though this can change over time, as do other aspects of their lives.

Two Viewing Requirements: Your Libido and Your Remote

Just as with any other sex toy, it helps if you're aroused before you begin watching porn. When you're ready to put the tape in and press "play," be sure to have the following items ready: lube, dildo, vibrator, towel, or all of the above, plus the remote control. Having a sex toy ready if you need it is handy because if the video turns you on and you want to get off, you won't have to interrupt it to search around for your toys.

But why the remote control? It's the only really required item for porn viewing: You'll need to fast forward through anything you don't like, or whatever distracts you from your arousal—be it lame dialogue, a sex act you don't care for, or a performer who turns you off. For some people this may seem like a hassle at first—why, you ask, can't the industry just make the "perfect" porn video?

The makers of porn try to appeal to as many tastes as possible in a relatively short amount of production time. Porn has to get to the point pretty quickly to retain horny viewers looking for instant gratification, and so, as in Hollywood, the folks who make porn have boiled down the content into formulas based on what they think viewers want.

Fun for Couples

Adding a lover to the festivities opens up a world of erotic possibilities. For many women, their first porn-watching experience is with a sweetheart, and if it's enjoyable at all, it's *really* enjoyable. Before you even start the tape, the air is charged with the foreknowledge that you're both about to so something naughty, fun, and highly sexual together, and this is a huge turn-on for many couples. Lots of couples like the whole ritual of renting (or buying) a tape, setting the scene, and watching together—it's a powerful aphrodisiac for two.

When you pick out a couple of tapes that you both are excited about, you each may have your own ideas about what you expect to happen—or what you *hope* to happen. Mostly sex, but how that sex happens is up to your individual desires. You might want to just use the tape as a little inspiration, to get turned on and have sex while the tape rolls.

One or both of you might have specific ideas about how the sex might progress, such as acting out what happens onscreen. He might hope she'll go down on him while he watches the movie, and she might want him to do the same. And there's no reason you can't do both! One of you might have had in mind a particular sex act that you've hoped will be introduced into your sex life—then, by a miracle, you see it on the tape! If this is you, then don't just sit there—make your desires heard. Your lover isn't a mind reader, and though porn is possibly the best conversation starter about sex, you'll have to indicate verbally at some point that you like what you see and want to try it yourself.

How to Talk About Porn with a Partner

When it comes to couples watching porn together, chances are high that one of you has the idea first, and must introduce the idea into the relationship. Some are lucky and find their lovers equally curious about the possible aphrodisiac effects of porn on their shared sex life, and look forward to trying something new that could really spice things up. Many who are introducing this new idea to novice porn viewers will receive a mixed reply—part curiosity, part apprehension. A few folks will be met with a reluctance to talk about it, while others might meet an outright refusal.

Either way, for you to explore the idea together, one of you has to be the one to start talking about it—easy if you talk about sex and experimentation regularly in your relationship, daunting if you never talk about sex, or porn. Not everyone has seen porn before, so it's possible that you're reading this book wanting to watch porn with a lover for your—or their—first time. Also, a significant number of people have watched porn and not enjoyed it, and they're apprehensive about trying again—unaware that there are literally hundreds of different types of adult videos available. But whatever your situation, telling your sweetie you want to try watching adult videos together can seem scary. Talking to your partner about sex can feel stressful. In fact, even thinking about talking about sex is stressful sometimes! If you've never brought up the subject of sex with your partner, don't worry. If you have what you consider a routine style of sex, telling your partner that you want something to change is scary, and starting a conversation about your desires to watch porn might make you feel extremely vulnerable—especially if you already watch porn on your own time, or used to watch it before your relationship. Opening yourself up and asking for something you want sexually takes courage and also gives you an opportunity to learn more about what your lover likes and dislikes.

If you don't normally talk about sex in your relationship and then suddenly one of you wants to watch an adult video, it might be upsetting—at first. Your lover may wonder if you've had sexual secrets all along. But it's very likely that your opening up this deliciously erotic Pandora's box will give them the opportunity to tell you what's on their mind about sex, too.

Before you begin, think about how you might bring up the subject in a way that would feel safe for you: You might feel more comfortable renting a mainstream movie with a slightly explicit sex scene in it (some suggestions are in the next section), and commenting on the scene. Or do you think you'd feel okay asking your partner what they think about porn while you're entwined in an intimate cuddle? Another technique you can try is telling them you want to confess a fantasy—a sexual one—and that he or she isn't to reply right away. Tell them that you can have a conversation about it later; this gives both of you time to let the idea settle.

Consider ways in which you can encourage your partner to hear you out, and ask them to suspend judgment until you can explain why this is important, and how good this new sexual behavior is going to make you feel—and be sure to reassure them that you find them incredibly sexy. The most important thing to think through beforehand is how you are going to make your partner feel safe when talking about it. Mentally rehearse what you'd like to say before you actually have the conversation. Think through possible scenarios, and imagine how they might react, so that you will be prepared to flow with whichever route the discussion might take.

NC-17 and Soft-Core Porn

If you or your lover don't feel ready to take the hard-core plunge, there are plenty of options that will still titillate the two of you. You can pick a Hollywood or foreign film that has an NC-17 rating, which is essentially a soft "X" and is either sought out by filmmakers for publicity or considered the "kiss of death" to features that hope to pull in the mainstream megabucks. European and Japanese films have fewer restrictions on sex and have a more mature, savvy viewership (not to mention legislators), so you'll find, say, French films with sex that doesn't hide—or exaggerate— real interactions. Or you can rent a soft-core feature, either a B-grade film with male and female nudity (no erections) or one with simulated sex. The *Red Shoe Diaries* series is the best-known of these films, largely for the appearance of David Duchovny in several episodes. Or you can watch cable TV or pay-per-view porn. Cable porn is softer than "hard core"—the stuff that shows penetration—though it's very similar because these films are the edited or softened version of a fully explicit porn feature. They show no penetration or genital close-ups—but it's definitely not simulated sex!

If you want to try out some steamy Hollywood or foreign movies, try these Hollywood pickin's:

Basic Instinct (director's cut)
Better Than Chocolate
Body of Evidence
Boogie Nights
Bound
Crash (director's cut)
The Fluffer
Henry and June
Holy Smoke
The Hunger
Jade
Kama Sutra
Last Tango in Paris
9 ½ Weeks
Secretary (highly recommended)

Soft-core or "soft porn" suggestions:
Cabin Fever
Emmanuelle
History of the Blue Movie
The Hottest Bid
Revelations
Score
The Story of O

Foreign:
Belle du Jour
Betty Blue
Emmanuelle
Fanny Hill
Hammer horror vampire films circa 1970
In the Realm of Passion
In the Realm of the Senses
Lesbian vampire films by Jess Franco or Jean Rollin
The Pillow Book
Romance
Sex and Lucia
Tokyo Decadence
The Unbearable Lightness of Being
Y Tu Mama Tambien

When Your Lover Is Reluctant

If your lover wants to try something sexually that you're afraid of or unsure about, or feel morally at question with, it can bring up powerful feelings. Adding any new sexual behavior to a relationship can feel like a make-or-break situation, and sometimes it is. Asking to try styles of expressing sexual intimacy can push your relationship to higher levels, or it can bring up so many issues that it rocks the boat—sometimes a little too hard. And porn touches on many issues that can be intense.

For many reasons, you or your lover may not want to watch porn. Understanding these concerns and hesitations can be helpful in having a constructive discussion about porn, learning how to overcome fears that might hold them back, and resolving what to do when one person does feel okay about watching porn yet the other doesn't. Or, if you're reading this book for yourself, you might learn how to set your concerns aside so that you can enjoy porn purely for the sole pleasure of getting yourself off.

The number one fear or concern people have about watching porn is that they won't stack up, or measure up, to the people they see onscreen. And whether they personally are comparing themselves to stars or starlets, or are worried that their lover might, they're right. After all, the people in porn look and act nothing like regular human beings.

Sure, they walk, they can talk (mostly), some can even snap their gum and have sex at the same time—and several have degrees in subjects such as entomology or microbiology and have very high IQs. But porn actors don't look anything like you or me, and that's why they got the job. Like Hollywood stars, porn stars are overblown caricatures of contemporary culture's ideals, and inhabit the tiny end of the gene pool. The actors are all very limber, and can withstand extended periods of sex in difficult positions under hot lights. They shave their balls, wax their asses, and sometimes wear makeup on virtually every inch of their bodies...and still perform. They can have sex with total strangers and make it look like it's not a job. It's *not* an easy job every day, but many actors make it look like pleasure.

Porn is fantasy, porn is fiction—even though the people up there having sex are flesh and blood. The films are heavily edited to make the sex last seemingly forever, to only show everyone's good angles, and to make the sex look like more than it is. Everyone appears to be having a good day—no PMS, no stress, no wrinkles, no headaches, and definitely no flaws, fat, or disabilities. No one gets pregnant from unsafe sex, or gets an STD. Men are always turned on and stay hard forever. Women seem to have orgasms from the slightest stimulation. Bodies, sexual response, sexual situations, and physical sex acts are not shown realistically in porn.

But still, we can't help but compare ourselves to the people we see onscreen. Porn can bring up a whole range of body issues, from feelings of inadequacy over small tits and dicks to worrying about your weight; from feeling ashamed of your vulva to wanting to hide the hair on your butt or back and the adult acne we all periodically fight. Porn, like Miss America contests, nudie magazines, television advertising, and music videos, can make us feel insecure about our desirability. It's also normal to worry that you or your lover might expect your sex lives to become like the sex you see onscreen, though this is unrealistic. Remember, porn actors are up there because they look different than everyone else and are willing to change their bodies (sometimes frightfully radically) to fit a fantasy "ideal." However, I think that precisely because it's so far away from reality, often the industry's purported "ideal" isn't what actually turns most of us on.

You might be worried that your lover will think porn stars are sexier than you are. Remember, porn isn't what we're supposed to be like. If you feel comfortable enough, tell your partner that you're worried about fitting into a fantasy ideal. You can always do some nonjudgmental poking around and ask your partner why he or she wants to watch porn, and then hear your partner out. Chances are good you'll hear it's because it turns your partner on, or might turn *you* on. Let your partner know that you want to stay their number one fantasy fuck.

Comparisons, judgments, and fear of the unfamiliar aside, the nervous porn virgin might have other worries as well. He or she might worry about seeing something offensive or disgusting that will be a turnoff—or worse. The chances of this are high in a film genre with the sole purpose of showing, in as much detail as possible, the vivid and explicit act of sex—a topic that is already difficult for some folks to explore. Listen to your partner's concerns, find out what he or she considers offensive, and tell them your concerns, too. Remember to include the judicious use of the remote control in your discussion, letting your partner know that you can fast-forward through anything he or she dislikes, or turn off the TV altogether and do something else if he or she would prefer. And try to inject a very necessary sense of humor about porn into your discussion. This is, after all, the film genre that brings you such titles as *Bat Dude and Throbbin, Shaving Ryan's Privates,* and *Terrors from the Clit.*

Watching Together

Introducing your partner to a new sex toy can be fun, and once you've come to the decision to watch together you have many fun ways to get the party started. The limits are your imagination, but here are a few suggestions:

• Together, read the review sections of this book, a catalog that features adult video reviews, or a website with reviews. It's a huge turn-on, and you can make a hot shopping list together.

• Venture together into the adult rental section of your local video store or a store that exclusively carries adult products. You don't have to get anything the first time out, but you can if it excites you both.

• If you both find a video or videos that you think might be fun, make a date, complete with dressing up and making a whole night of it. This can be a good way to deemphasize the viewing—helpful for nervous partners and downplaying the effects of a potentially disappointing film.

• With a film you both want to watch, make a special surprise out of it. Mail it to them with a love note indicating a date to watch together, or slip it under their pillow, or wrap it up and present it as dessert after a romantic dinner.

Sex While You Watch

You can have sex in a variety of ways, as the video plays onscreen, or not have sex at all and save your excitement for later. Here are suggestions for watching with a lover:

- Try out the positions of the actors onscreen, following along with the action.
- Use positions that make watching easy for both of you. Try a reverse lap straddle ("reverse cowgirl"), or spooning facing the TV, or lying face-to-face but facing the screen.
- Doggie-style works well if you have enough room. Incorporate extra furniture as props for comfort or easing injuries and mobility issues. A hassock or padded footstool can make doggie-style effortless for the recipient.
- Take turns watching while one person performs oral sex on the other.
- Watch with your hands in each other's laps under a blanket.

One alternative is to view the film in its entirety and have sex afterward. More than one couple I surveyed for this book claimed that after they watched a porn movie that both parties thought was awful or boring, they had supercharged sex when the TV was off. Perhaps they were stimulated by explicit images, period, or felt like they had to show each other what genuinely hot sex was really like!

You don't have to be entirely consumed by the movie to use it to enhance your sex life. Instead of the film as the main focus, use it as a prop or tool:

- Try playing a tape for your lover to watch in one room as you dress (or undress) for sex in the next room—talk about getting ready!
- Have a tape running in the background with the sound off for extra visual stimulation as you seduce your lover with a lap dance or massage.
- Be watching the video when they get home from work and pretend to be "caught in the act."

Couples who enjoy more advanced sex styles, such as BDSM or role-playing, can use porn to their advantage in a number of ways. Folks who are used to employing negotiation, consent, and all the highly creative trappings of power-play in their sexual relationships will already have an arsenal of ideas about how to use virtually anything to torture and titillate their lovers, though here I offer a few ideas as well:

- If you're dominant, tie your (willing) lover to a chair where he or she "must" watch the movie. You can also instruct your partner not to move or speak…or else.
- While he or she watches a video, have your way with him or her. Use your lover as a sex toy as you enjoy the video.
- With bondage, the restrained party can be erotically tortured while the film runs, heightening his or her arousal.
- Have your partner view an entire video without being allowed to touch himself or herself.
- Tell your partner the movie the two of you are about to watch is what will happen when the tape is over. Then do it.
- Comfortably watch and enjoy the film as your partner "services" you.
- If you both like to switch roles, one can be tied down to watch the video as the other orally services the bound participant.
- If you enjoy S/M, you can add to the feel of your "dungeon" by having an S/M tape running in the background for ambiance as you enact your own scene.
- Role-playing along with the tape is a lot of fun. Maybe your honey is a "bad girl" like the one in the video!

Porn Sex Games

Watching arousing videos together is fun all on its own, but since variation is the spice of life, try any of these porn sex games to turn up the heat.

Give Me a Kiss

This game is very similar to movie "drinking games" where everyone imbibes an alcoholic beverage in response to a repetitive onscreen activity—but this game intoxicates only your libido. Every time an actor onscreen says, "oh god," "oh yeah," "fuck, yeah," or "yeah yeah yeah," the fastest one to repeat the dialogue gets to kiss the other one on any part of his or her body—and can even direct the slowpoke to reciprocate.

Variation: The slow one must sexually mimic whatever the actor's counterpart is doing onscreen.

S/M Variation: When the dialogue is spoken onscreen, the dominant partner gets to pinch, spank, bite, or clamp a clothespin on the submissive—as the intensity of the dialogue increases, so does the pain (and everyone's pleasure).

Head of the Class

This one requires unheard-of self restraint, but the results are well worth the wait. Watch an entire video without touching yourselves, or each other. When the video is over, write down a list of your favorite parts, or things you wish you had seen in the film. Trade lists for later play.

Variation: You can watch the video on your own time and then slip the report to your lover in public, or somewhere equally naughty.

My Favorite Chair

Talk about a thrill ride! Flip a coin. "Heads" gets to be the "chair." With the partner sitting on the "chair's" lap, the "chair" is free to explore the sitter's body while both enjoy the movie. Switch at each scene. This game works best with an all-sex video.

Any Game Will Do

The next time you play pinball, Ping-Pong, horseshoes, golf, poker, or any other game, make it the hottest you ever played. You can cash in on these sexy high stakes when you get home and pop your favorite porn film into the DVD player:

Secret Shopper: The winner gets to select an adult video to watch together.

Be My Pornstar: The loser must act out the winner's favorite scene from an adult video.

Remote Control: One wins control of the remote for the duration of a sex scene, or an entire video.

Bound Bliss: One is tied to a chair and made to watch porn, while the winner has free hands to roam and enjoy themselves—and every inch of their bound subject.

Sex Toy Tease: The winner gets a sex toy to play with while the other is forbidden to use even their hands.

Surprise Buzz: Using remote controlled vibrating panties, butt plugs, or even simply vibrators with a long cord, the winner controls the other's vibration according to their whims.

Selecting a Tape for Your Lover

Renting or buying a movie for someone else isn't easy, unless you know the person quite well and have an intuitive feel for their likes and dislikes. I can't count the number of times I have had a friend tell me to go see a movie in the theaters, or lend me a copy of their favorite Hollywood film to watch, and been utterly disappointed or outright confused that the person I thought was my really smart friend would like such dreck. But I shrug it off and think "to each his own," and tell my friend thanks anyway. This situation is even more acute when it comes to porn.

With adult movies, you're seeking to suit not only your lover's tastes in film, but also the whole complex world of their sexual likes and dislikes. Unless you know for sure that your partner likes films by Seymore Butts or videos with Rocco in them, you're playing a guessing game in which you need to be part detective and part intuitive sleuth. If you put some thought and research into your selections, the rewards will be many.

Your first step is to familiarize yourself with porn. Learn the subgenres and the context in which the sex acts are presented. Then think about what he or she likes and dislikes in both movies and sex. Reflect on any comments you might have heard your friend make about XXX films, how actresses and actors look, or porn in general. Does this person think fake boobs are icky? Does he or she like it when sex is depicted roughly, or not rough at all, or very softly? Does he or she especially like a partic-ular sex act, such as anal sex or blow jobs? Have you heard your friend or partner mention that he or she would like to watch porn, if only it were like a regular Hollywood film?

Cultivate an idea of what you think this person might enjoy before you go to the video store, and make a list of prospective titles or types of films. If you go to a woman-owned sex toy store, you'll have a good chance of being able to talk to a friendly and knowledgeable staff mem-ber who can point you in the right direction. But if you don't live near a major city, where most of these stores are located, you're on your own, so go armed with as much information as you can. Make some selections from this book before you make your commitment, and pick videos with icons that indicate the kind of performers, attention to female pleasure (especially if your partner is female), and high production values—or whatever else you might like.

Ideally, the best thing to do is to go to the store or browse a website with the person with whom you're going to watch the tape. But if it's a gift, surprise, or planned event in which you are the lucky courier, consider renting more than one title. Renting tapes is the ideal scenario, because if you get something they don't like you're not out $40 or $50. This isn't an option for everyone, though many websites do rent porn online.

For the first-time viewer, even porn with high values and a plot might seem awkward and cheesy compared to the average TV show or movie. If you're not sure your partner will like porn, but you still want to test the waters, consider renting either a soft-core film or a highly sexual Hollywood film that got an NC-17 rating. Make your big leap together into the world of explicit onscreen sex a hot, fun-filled adventure—together!

CHAPTER

3

Get the Porn You Want

*I like it when we leave the video store, and she's
carrying the X-rated videos!*

Finding the tape—or DVD—that turns you on and gets you
off is no easy proposition, even if you already know what
you want to see. Adult film is a vast genre with many subgenres, full of its own language and customs, confusing
labels, and misleading titles—plus a whole lot of bad
grammar. What's worse, many retailers treat their stock
with carelessness or even distaste, cramming rooms full of
video and DVD boxes with no discernable sense of order.
Alphabetical order is not invited to the party, Dewey deci-
mal has left the building. It's a little easier on the Web,
but still each site seems to have its own organizational logic.
It would make a librarian homicidal.

In a lot of ways, finding the adult tape you want to rent or buy is much like seeking out a Hollywood movie—you're really on your own to find it. But in a genre of film that has no road map, you'll need to know not only what you want and where to find it, but also the different types of porn available.

Start Here

Begin by going over your personal laundry lists of what you want to see and what you hope to avoid. Read the reviews in this book to help get your ideas together, as well as to give you a sense of what's available. You may discover something you didn't know about, something that you find sexually interesting. You might also find something that turns you off, or that you don't care to see at all. Be prepared for the inevitable: No matter how open-minded you are, you will at some point come across a box cover, turn of phrase, or scene in an adult video that will offend you. Just because it's out there doesn't mean you ever have to have it in your life for more than that fleeting instant.

Create a picture of what you hope to find in a video as you would order a meal in a restaurant. What things turn you on? Small breasts, big butts, women in charge, realistic plots, blow jobs, two gals and a guy, male anal penetration, rough sex? This may not be *your* list, but you get the idea. The important thing is that you make a list of all the qualities you hope to find in an adult film. Then make a second list of things you *don't* want to see. Do you get turned off by fake breasts, hairy men, rimming, toe-sucking, facial ejaculation, two women together, or watching group sex? These are just examples to get you brainstorming about what you think will send you over the edge—and what you think you'll want to fast-forward through. As you watch porn, you'll probably find more to add to either list, because sometimes we find things that turn us on or off that we didn't even know about.

For instance, you might want a movie with no plot, all-natural women, authentic female orgasms, and no men. Or maybe you want a great story line and believable acting, and you don't care what anyone looks like as long as the sex is hot. Perhaps you want an S/M film that looks beautiful, with no plot and with real couples. Maybe you want a lesbian love story but no genital close-ups. You might be fantasizing about a specific type of story, where the women are the main focus, but you don't want anal penetration. Or you want all-anal, as rough as it gets.

The choices are many, and the selection is vast. You might not be able to find exactly the film you're looking for, but you'll find a lot that come arousingly close. To help narrow your wish list into a set of realistic parameters, learn porn's categories by reading the next chapter. These will help you nail down specifics, such as the type of sex act, how it's presented, the film style, the kind of people in the films, and for what audience the video's intended. And learning the categories is the perfect place to start learning adult video terminology.

Renting and Buying

Renting is the most economical choice when watching adult films. This way, you can test the water with a $3–$5 rental before jumping in with an investment of $30 or more. Renting, though, isn't always a convenient option for everyone. If you must buy, you'll want to make your video and retailer choices carefully. Check the Resources, Chapter 14, for recommendations on stores, mail-order retailers, and websites where you can purchase privately and with confidence.

Your best bet for rentals is your local video store or local adult store. In your regular video store, they likely have a room or area sectioned off from the rest of the store that is for adults only. Some stores keep their video box covers in giant books for customers to leaf through; if your store doesn't appear to have any adult videos, then look for a book or ask if they carry adult videos. They'll keep the book behind the counter, away from young eyes.

Before you make your rental trip, take a fact-finding mission to the video store first, so that you don't become overwhelmed by all the assaulting box covers with their explicit photos, attention-grabbing titles, and utter lack of order. Check it out, and plan to rent on your second trip. On your maiden rental trip, have a checklist in your mind of what you want—movie titles, actors, directors, series, or sex acts. Making an actual list is very helpful. Don't go in the store for one video only, in case they don't have it or it's checked out—be prepared to be versatile.

It takes a conscious effort to enter the hard-core section for the first time, and if you're female, be prepared for men who were browsing before you came in to flee. I kind of like it—I get the section to myself. But just ignore everyone else, and help yourself to what is rightfully yours as an adult. If you decide to go to an adults-only store where you'll have a better selection, men may not flee, but you might be the only woman in sight. Then again, you could be surprised to see other women and couples shopping for porn and sex toys. It's happening more and more every year.

If your town has one of the nation's many warm, welcoming, women-friendly sex toy stores, don't hesitate to shop there for your adult videos and DVDs, with the aid of the knowledgeable staff that run the registers. The workers in these stores typically know a lot about the videos they carry and can point you in the right direction. Your first experience in one of these "clean, well-lit" places to shop for sex toys and videos will be a shock—no sleaze! Many of these stores are designed and run like upscale boutiques, but without the cheesy element of "novelty" adult stores. The women-friendly shops focus on educating their customers about the products and promote a woman-oriented approach to sexual pleasure, and have hand-picked selections of the best videos they can find—usually reviewed and prescreened in-house by female video reviewers. As a customer, you'll be joining the (literally) millions of other women and men shopping in these stores—people of every stripe and persuasion, having fun renting and buying adult videos, and also purchasing vibrators, cock rings, and other sex toys. Unfortunately, these terrific shops are found only in a few major cities. San Francisco and Berkeley (Good Vibrations), Seattle (Toys in Babeland), Austin (Forbidden Fruit), Boston and Los Angeles (Grand Opening), New York (Toys in Babeland), Toronto (Come as You Are, Good for Her), and other cities have women-friendly sex toy shops.

If you don't happen to live near one of these retailers, and have limited Internet access, look in your local phone book for adult stores under the headings "Video Tapes & Discs–Sales & Rentals," or look for the adults-only section in your usual local video rental store. Most major cities have a selection of adult toy, book, and video shops that are somewhat (or even very) sleazy and uncomfortable to shop in, generally because they aren't clean or kept up in any visible way, and the customers and clerks don't seem to want to be seen there. However, not all adult shops are like this, and some will have female staff, witty gay clerks, or an owner who works behind the counter and has a wealth of knowledge to share— even if it's just knowing on which shelf to find a particular title. Some of the low-end video stores have an "arcade" in the back, where men pay to "test drive" the videos. This is a little unsettling for those who aren't familiar with this culture, and many women might feel worried about going into a store with an arcade. The best way to handle this is to march right in during daylight hours, bringing a friend or two and ignoring every-one else. But believe me, after years of going into every kind of adult video rental store imaginable doing research for this book, if you're a woman and you go into one of the seedier shops, I'll bet cash money that you'll be the only one in the store within two minutes. Our culture is so packed with sexual shame that whenever I walk into an arcade to find a video, the men run for cover, leaving me free to take my time shopping for my next rental.

The local mom-and-pop video stores will have a closed back room where they keep the adult videos and DVDs, away from the tender eyes of those under 18. As mentioned earlier, some stores opt to save on space and will have their adult video selection in large books that are kept behind the counter, containing box covers in a sort of big flipbook. If you don't see an annex for adult videos, or a room with western-style swing doors, ask to see their adult video books. Expect that the adult titles will be more expensive than what you usually pay for a rental—these videos are much more likely not to be returned than their other videos, and retailers like to have insurance against losing their stock (hence the higher prices).

You might wind up going to more than one store to find what you want, or a place where you feel comfortable shopping. You don't have to settle for the first place, or the nearest store, if you don't like it—remember, *you're the customer*. If you look around, you'll find what you're looking for, and if you have a particular title in mind you can always call ahead to see if they have it; some stores will set titles aside for regular customers.

Privacy and discretion are two main concerns for adult video shoppers. You can choose to peruse stores away from your home and work. Or go rent your videos when the store isn't busy, like on a weekday. You can have your lover rent for you—make it an erotic "command" if you like. Or you can just not give a damn what anyone thinks about your private sex life. And don't concern yourself with what the person behind the counter thinks about you, unless they're being inappropriate, of course. They've seen it all before, and they're probably worrying about theft, or register balances, or the various problems porn store clerks contend with.

Going into an actual store is really the best way to shop, and some people even go to the women-friendly shops to look at the toys and videos, and then order online from the privacy of their own homes. But since going into a local, friendly shop is not an option for everyone, many people choose to buy and rent their adult videos and DVDs through mail order or the Internet. If discretion is an issue for you, then the Internet is your friend. The privacy that the Internet affords has made it both easy and safe for everyone to try out new sexual ideas and explore new possibilities, plus it puts adult videos within everyone's reach. The Internet's drawback is that ordering and renting videos can be dicey if you don't know the company's privacy policy (some companies sell your information to other parties), and it's more difficult to ask questions about the videos. Be aware that any catalog you order from the back of a magazine will be through a third-party source—not directly from the magazine publisher itself—and this third party will sell your address to other businesses. But all the online resources listed in this book have their privacy policies on their websites, and many of them even have customer reviews on individual titles. Sometimes these reviews are lengthy, making it easy for you to make a clear decision that includes the sex acts and performers you want to see but excludes the stuff that turns you off. Additionally, some sites are dedicated to reviews, with links to sites where you can rent or buy titles—how convenient!

Renting or purchasing online is an easy, private, and simple way to find and obtain the videos or DVDs you're looking for. Some people find it a big pain to deal with the organizational chaos of finding stores and wasting travel time (including parking, in big cities) merely to rent porn in person, and are overjoyed to find that online transactions have quieted these complaints. Purchasing online is as simple as buying a book, and renting is just as painless, though each online store has its own policies and rules about rentals. For a list of recommended online rental and purchase sites, see "Resources," Chapter 14.

Renting an adult video or DVD online sounds a little strange if you've never tried it before. But sites that offer these wares are usually the best resources for finding and selecting what you want. They typically have excellent search engines, allowing you to search by title, director, actor, or genre (such as lesbian, heterosexual, or bisexual), and sometimes by studio, such as VCA or Evil Angel. They cater to a smorgasbord of tastes and sexual orientations, and might have suggestions that help turn up tasty selections for you. Then, you make your choice by clicking the "rent" button, at which time the site will drop that item into your virtual shopping cart and allow you to shop for another video. Online renters usually limit how many videos and DVDs you can select—up to three is standard, but some go up to eight—plus a time limit for how long you can hold onto them. Most sites will let you hold your selection video while you shop for up to an hour, but then return the video to the "shelves" so others can shop for it, too. When ready to check out, you set up an account with a required credit card, and pay for your rentals. Each company has a different rental pricing structure; some are per rental, while others have a flat monthly fee. The rentals are shipped to you discreetly—these businesses want your return patronage!—and you keep the videos for a set number of days, usually seven (a full week). The rentals arrive typically within a few business days, and include a return envelope with postage. You watch the videos as many times as you like, then drop them in the mail when you're done.

DVD vs. VHS Tapes: Making Porn Better?

Because we are constantly barraged with ads about what's just around the corner for the next generation of cell phones, or how the next Palm Pilot is going to bring you the paper and your slippers on Sunday mornings, it's easy to get cynical about what's new and useful in the marketplace. I remember a great TV commercial depicting a man driving in a convertible and looking all smug about his new purchase—a computer strapped into the passenger seat, the "H-6." As he drove by a billboard, workers were already pasting up a new ad for the "H-7," wiping the smile right off our once-sated consumer's face. Which points to some people's hesitations about new tech, including the push to make a switch from VHS (for "Video Home System") to DVD (for "Digital Video Disc" or "Digital Versatile Disc")—raising many questions as to why we might do such a thing. Especially from the perspective of a porn consumer.

For the people who are already DVD porn consumers, "DVD vs. VHS?" is a moot question. In their minds, the benefits of DVD porn far outweigh the plusses of the old VHS format for porn. What bears examining is the way porn is used as a sex toy, and how that applies to the interface for the user. People use porn to get off in a variety of ways, but in general there are two kinds of viewers: One enjoys being pulled into a story line or visual world, being aroused by a variety of fantasy imagery; the other relishes their visual sex straight, no chaser (so to speak), and wants to view a particular sex act for instant fantasy-fuel and release. The one wants to receive fantasy from an outside source, while the other has a predetermined fantasy they want to see acted out—and this equates to watching plot-driven porn or all-sex, no-story porn.

For the all-sex crowd, DVDs are ideal. Say you want to get off watching one sex act (like cunnilingus), a particular part of the sex act (like a facial come shot), a specific fantasy scenario (a guy with one woman on his face and another going down on him), or sex with a certain actor or actress. With VHS, you need to watch the whole tape to get to the scene you want to see. Then, when you find the scene, you masturbate and rewind repeatedly until you see enough of the scene to reach orgasm—a scenario that is frustrating, rife with opportunity for operator error, and difficult to time with your orgasm. Believe me, it can be done, but the effort often outweighs the enjoyment of the resulting orgasm.

With a DVD, the all-sex viewer can avoid many of these frustrations. The person who wants to jump right to a particular scene with one actor or actress can first view the menu, with an overview of all scenes broken down into "chapters," and go directly to the scene they want to see. Looking for a specific sex act is much easier, as some DVD players have "jog/shuttle" on their remotes, making moving around the disc a breeze. On all DVD players, the viewer can fast-forward and rewind at multiple speeds, from slow to super-fast, and the picture is crystal-clear, so you don't miss any subtleties when searching for that one thing that gets you off. Some players even have zoom functions, allowing the viewer to examine certain elements of a scene in greater detail, and even play picture and sound while zoomed in. And for repeating the sequence you like, most of the new, even the inexpensive, players have what's called an "A–B" function, or "repeat from point A to point B," that lets you program the player to show a specific segment (whether a few seconds or many minutes or segments) over and over, until you're done—hands free.

Viewers who like to sink into the story and enjoy the seduction of a well-shot, carefully constructed porn film will find that DVDs take their viewing style even further. In this case, the bonuses are in the DVDs themselves, rather than the DVD player. The first thing to notice is the unbelievably crisp, clear picture—and I'll admit that once you see the remarkable picture from a DVD, you won't want to settle for less again (further, viewing a DVD film on an HDTV is like watching a clear 3-D picture, but without those annoying red/blue glasses). The sound quality is amazing too, though this feature is seldom a plus in porn, where sound quality is usually poor and the sound tracks often lame. Some DVDs, however, allow the user to eliminate the sound track altogether, eliminate dialogue, or offer options to hear the director or an actor's commentary throughout the film. Some porn DVDs offer true multiple angles, allowing the viewer to "virtually" move the camera around to watch from different angles. And many offer other pluses after the feature, such as extra scenes, interviews with stars and directors, slide shows of the best scenes, porn bloopers, alternate endings, outtakes, and more—all of which you can skip to by using the menu at any time.

Those who like a good story with their plot will also appreciate DVDs' system of "chapters," where scenes or plot points are broken down on the main menu. If you have to stop viewing for any reason, you can eject the disc and come back later to the specific point in the story that you left, simply by selecting that chapter from the menu.

Also, if you find a film that you really like, DVDs will outlast VHS tapes, barring any surface scratches to the disc. VHS tapes stretch, get eaten in VCRs, can lose their magnetic charge over time, and are fallible by virtue of their clunky design. By contrast, the DVD is wafer-thin, strong, and not susceptible to getting mashed by (or stuck in) tape rollers. However, not all porn films are available on DVD, so you may need to seek out the old reliable VHS versions of some classics, independents, fetish-specific, or difficult-to-find videos. But combination DVD/CD players have come down so much in price—they cost the same as or less than a new VCR (they're much cheaper to manufacture)—that many distributors are rushing to get as many movies onto that medium as they can to cash in, before DVDs plummet further in price. It has become much easier and cheaper to rent DVDs as well, much easier in fact than VHS tapes. Many of the garden-variety adult stores dropped their DVD rental prices right after the 2002–2003 holiday season, from the cost of a new VHS rental (for non-new releases) to the same cost as a regular VHS rental. Websites that rent and sell DVD porn have sprung up like mushrooms after a rain, operating the same way as other DVD rental sites, making DVD selection and rental fantastically easy. Gone are the worries about late fees and venturing into adult stores, not to mention whether they'll have your tape or not. Now you can browse an online selection in the privacy of your home, do research on a particular title and read reviews, then rent online, have the discs sent to you, and drop them in the mail when you're done. Each site has its own policies regarding price and rental rules, but most sites are incredibly economical, and you can go to any store online you want with the click of a mouse.

While I once was a hardened tech skeptic, now I have to say that with DVD, porn is a better sex toy. And getting off better is the bottom line.

What's on the Box

When you're considering a video or DVD hands-on, look closely at the box or case. Check for the names you're looking for, or for ones you want to avoid. Look at the teeny-tiny pictures—these will be stills taken during the filming of the video. You can see right off the bat if there's anything you don't like. Sometimes you'll see pictures of scenes or actresses on the box that aren't in the video, though this is happening less frequently as consumer outcry makes pornographers begin to guarantee that images on the box actually come from the video itself. By all means, don't get a video with an offensive title, subtitle, or image. Get a video you'll feel okay about watching, whether or not you get off.

Box covers in porn are glossy, colorful, and very eye-catching—and usually sexually explicit. Higher-budget films will have a big, fancy, professionally retouched photo on the front cover, with the star or stars looking way more packaged than they will in the actual film. All-sex features have a couple of collaged images on the cover, as a sample of the performers inside (usually the more conventionally beautiful ones), with small images of the explicit action around them as window dressing. These small images might be slightly censored or nonexplicit. Other genres will have a range of covers, from the high-budget style (looks like an ordinary movie) to the low-budget (cramming in as many pics as possible). The box cover backs will have many more tiny explicit photos—look at these eye-straining photos closely, and you'll have a pretty good idea of what's in the video. In the high-budget features, the layout might be more like a regular movie box, with a small descriptive blurb about the feature and the sex acts and perhaps a short review or endorsement from an adult video magazine.

The text on the box covers will range from hilarious to offensive, from artsy to unintelligible and error-ridden. The words can be so misspelled and ungrammatical that you won't know whether you want to laugh or weep openly for the public school system. Still, the description, however haphazard, will give you an idea about what you'll find inside. In all-sex films, it's a good idea to look for boxes that state that all images on the box cover depict scenes on the video (your seal of approval), or to stick with reputable companies or directors. For quality in features, look for well-known production houses, directors, and stars.

The Cambria List

In early 2001 *Adult Video News* reported on a list of guidelines for video box covers intended to protect adult filmmakers from legal scrutiny and obscenity charges. Some say that the list represents guidelines strictly for box covers and the sex acts they depict, while others feel that some of the guidelines should extend to the actual content of the videos. The tricky part is that while a video that shows someone urinating on a lover would be considered whitebread in a San Francisco video store, it would be thought obscene by community standards in rural Wyoming. Adult industry attorney Paul Cambria helped prepare the list, and while it is largely used as a set of rules by the mainstream heterosexual video companies, a few others aggressively mock the list with every video they produce. Talk about not seeing the forest for the trees! But when you read over the list you'll see some very confusing items, some very common fantasies, sex acts common in porn, and some unfortunate distancing from racial issues.
The list:

Box Cover Guidelines/Movie Production Guidelines

Before selecting a chrome please check facial expression. Do not use any shots that depict unhappiness or pain.
Do not include any of the following:
No: shots with appearance of pain or degradation, facials (bodyshots are OK if shot is not nasty), bukkake, spitting or saliva mouth to mouth, food used as sex object, peeing unless in a natural setting (e.g., field, roadside), coffins, blindfolds, wax dripping, two dicks in/near one mouth, shot of stretching pussy, fisting, squirting, bondage-type toys or gear unless very light, girls sharing same dildo (in mouth or pussy), hands from 2 different people fingering same girl, male/male penetration, transsexuals, bi-sex, degrading dialogue (e.g., "Suck this cock, bitch" while slapping

her face with a penis), menstruation topics, incest topics, forced sex, rape themes, etc., and no black men–white women themes. Toys are OK if shot is not nasty.

As you can see, sometimes these guidelines are followed, though they're often ignored by the majority of porn makers. Some pornographers deliberately set out to disobey the most extreme rules on the list, to the irritation of other filmmakers who want to exercise as much caution as possible to keep below censors' radar screens. But either way, you will wind up seeing a sample of what you're getting on the box cover. In a way, a filmmaker's disobeying these rules is just fine for the consumer—since, in many cases, the rules are ridiculous and don't apply either to porn's content or to what real consumers want to see. And when you see on the box cover what's in the actual video, you can make a selection that better fits your tastes.

Awards for Porn Films?

A video is more likely to have something in it worth watching if its box cover text touts any awards or honors it has garnered, such as an *AVN,* Hot d'Or, *Adam Film World,* or XRCO Choice (X-Rated Critics Organization) award. *AVN Magazine* and *Hot Video Magazine* both produce yearly awards events that bestow honors on worthy videos, crew, directors, and actors. Each of the events is a lavish production—big money, black-tie, haute couture, limo-packed. At these well-attended spectacles big stars show lots of skin, and plenty of lone guys flock to ogle and have their pictures taken with the stars in the off-hours of the events. The awards ceremonies themselves are steeped in tradition, last for ages, and serve dinner to the esteemed guests who paid hundreds of dollars a seat. The invitation-only parties are the prize, of course, and are legendary in their decadence.

Adult Video News is a magazine by and for the porn industry. The scope of *AVN* is wide-ranging, including everything from movie reviews by genre to free speech news and legal updates on censorship in America.

It's a slick, glossy magazine full of ads for the latest releases; industry gossip; news about stars, directors, and production houses; and reviews of adult books, comics, magazines, sex toys, S/M gear, and adult websites. *AVN* has a sprawling site, www.avn.com (beware of pop-ups), and spin-off magazines such as *AVN Online*. Every year in Las Vegas it holds an awards event where juries select from nominated films a whole roster of winners for a variety of categories, ranging from "Best New Starlet" and "Best Director" to "Best Fellatio Scene." Winning an award is a coveted prize, and can launch careers, boost sales, and make a film noticed by everyone. When you see an *AVN* award, you know you've got a good film in the can (or the digicam). *AVN* also has an all-gay-male version, the GayVN's. *AVN* also awards a Best European Film honor called the AVN d'Or.

The "Palme d'Or" is the highest award possible for a director to receive at Cannes, the celebrated international film festival held yearly in France. Held at the same time as Cannes, the Hot d'Or Awards celebrate European adult films, much like the *AVNs*. Produced by French magazine *Hot Video*, often called the French version of *AVN*, the decade-old event packs more than 500 people into a ballroom every year. They give a nod to America's porn industry with selective awards—though usually the general contenders for awards are half American, half European. In the jury process, few awards are actually selected by industry professionals—called the Professional Vote—and most are selected by *Hot Video's* readers.

Founded in 1985, the XRCO Awards are held every year in Century City, California. These awards are voted on by members of the adult print media as well as Internet critics, and though the ceremonies are much smaller and intimate, with little of the nonindustry throngs that clog up events like *AVN's*, the event is still piled high with pornerati glitz and glam. The XRCO is composed of the industry's top critics and reviewers from a wide range of adult publications, including *Adam Film World*, *AVN*, and *Hustler*, as well as Internet retail sites. *Adam Film World Guide* is an industry magazine that serves as a guide and hosts a readers' poll to select the award winners.

Many other erotic film festivals flourish around the world, such as the Barcelona Erotic Film Festival, the 18 Awards (in the UK), the New York City Erotic Film Fest, and more. However, few mainstream adult films are awarded at these events, so you won't see many box cover mentions with these names. Some independent adult films occasionally cause a stir at nonerotic independent film festivals, as did Maria Beatty's *The Black Glove*.

What's in a Name?

Adult video titles will make you laugh or cry, arouse you or make you want to run away screaming—sometimes all at once. The desperate namers try every possible crass (and clever) deviation on any remotely sexual saying, phrase, or nonerotic movie title. Although the titles can seem simultaneously idiotic, amusing, salacious, lowbrow, and lame, what the video is called can actually tell you quite a lot about the movie you're about to rent.

Many serial videos have no plot, and their title will tell you the main theme of the series. The obvious ones focus on a particular sex act, such as *Real Female Masturbation, Gush, Buttman's Big Tit Adventure, Blowjob Fantasies, Bend Over Boyfriend*—the list runs to infinity. Some series titles include a name that denotes a particular director's style, like Shane, Seymore Butts, Ben Dover, Ed Powers, and others. Many offer a stylistic theme, such as a film style, concept, or gimmick. The *Voyeur* series, for example, is seen through the eyes of a mysterious peeping tom and is the product of a single director, John Leslie. Each video in the *Deep Inside* series, for another example, focuses on the same actress; she gives a tour of her favorite scenes from all her films, which were shot by a number of directors.

Feature videos, or videos that have a plot (often a *very* loose term), will have names that are all over the map. The name depends on what the filmmaker wants to convey, and how much he cares—or doesn't care—about the product and the viewer. For quite a few pornographers, making porn is a subversive joke, and they'll name their videos accordingly. It should be noted, however, that the majority of pornographers

The Revenge of Edward Penishands

WHILE I CAN'T VOUCH FOR THE film quality of these titles, here is a sampling of some great adult spoof titles:

Ally McFeal
American Booty
The Bare Dick Project
Blowjob Impossible
Buffy the Vampire Layer
Cliffbanger
A Clockwork Orgy
Das Boob
Dude, Where's My Dildo?
Edward Penishands
Ejacula
Fast Times at Deep Crack High
Free Will Humping

Honey, I Blew Everybody
Howard Sperm's Private Parties
Juranal Park
Moulin Splooge
The Ozporns
Pimped by an Angel
Poltergash
Saturday Night Beaver
Shaving Ryan's Privates
Snatch Adams
The Sopornos
A Tale of Two Titties
Thighs Wide Open
Thunderboobs
Twin Cheeks
White Men Can't Hump
Whore of the Rings

don't seem to consider their audience to be very smart, and will think they're catering to—or making fun of—an uneducated, unsophisticated viewer who provides their bread and butter. On the flipside, many directors and producers do care about the end product as a living legacy, a video that will be seen by all types of people, and will therefore strive to make complete, even artistic films. One obstacle in porn is that it's tough to make a fully realized film when you have to include the same specific scenes in each video. Nonetheless, like the classics, features will have a variety of names: movie-like, smart, evocative, romantic, dumb, or hilarious.

Spoofs of mainstream movies or cult classics are the best-known titles in adult video culture, and sometimes they're really good spoofs. Usually, though, they're just a long running joke that never gets off the ground, and all you have is a porn film with actors trying to say lines with bad accents in costumes that would make a drag queen want to claw her own eyes out.

Finding what you want to see is still going to be somewhat trial-and-error, and you'll need to be open to the fact that you're on an ongoing, exciting search for hot porn. Your ideas and fantasies will be refined and shaped as you discover what sex acts you like, what type of performers you enjoy, and how you prefer to see them presented. Because our desires and fantasies are constantly changing, no one model of porn—such as all-sex or plot-only—is going to fulfill every visual fantasy you have at every period of your life. And because finding specific titles, directors, and actors is a constant challenge in a genre that is haphazardly maintained by retailers, you'll need to have a number of alternate choices ready when you go to the video store, sex toy store, or online retailer. For a complete list, consult the Resources, Chapter 14.

4

A Porn Primer

I like to make an event out of it: a good quality tape,
cued up to just the scene I want to see, lube, a sex
toy, and I'm off to multiple orgasm land.

When you bring home your first porn video or DVD, you may
expect to see a movie just like a mega-budget Hollywood
blockbuster, but one that goes "all the way" instead of fading out when the sex scene begins. In some porn films, you
will see a Hollywood standard of high production values—
they even "leave the lights on" when the sex begins—though
not all films are like this. Why not? Because outside
Hollywood studios, no one has that kind of money or those
resources to throw around, especially in a film genre that's
controversial.

Mainstream porn is like independent film, with the difference that the people behind and in front of the camera

haven't gone to school to learn and cultivate style and technique that we're used to seeing, since most folks in the industry didn't intend porn to be their first career choice. But what is truly remarkable is the large number of adult filmmakers who pull off amazing feats with virtually nothing—no budget, no time, untrained actors, and few resources. In the big business of making porn, it's the people at the top making all the distribution decisions (and all the money), while the people actually making the films—the actors, directors, and crew—are at the bottom of the financial food chain. If Hollywood could do what the adult industry directors, writers, actors, and crew do out of blood, sweat, and tears—and with the same hunger to fulfill a creative drive while making a pittance—we'd have a lot more films in theaters worth watching.

Mainstream and Independent Porn

Porn is a genre of film in its own right, with subgenres representing films that appeal to particular audiences or are made in a particular style. As in Hollywood, in porn there are mainstream films and independent films. The term *mainstream* indicates films made by the bigger companies like Vivid, VCA, Wicked, Metro, Adam and Eve, and Evil Angel (to name a few), largely based in Southern California. Mainstream porn films are the most widely available, usually featuring "typical" porn actors—all stars and of little diversity in terms of skin color, ethnic background, and body size. Mainstream studios put a lot of money into their films and keep some outstanding actors and directors in their stables.

Independent porn, by contrast, refers to films made by the little guys, and, as with nonadult independent movie studios, the genre boasts a lot of innovators and art school directors, who often are edgier and provide more realistic and thought-provoking content. Independently made porn comes from all over, though is largely based in the United States, and is made by individuals such as Maria Beatty (Bleu Productions), woman-owned production companies like SIR Video and Fatale, and small companies such as Libido Films (formerly *Libido Magazine*) and Sexpositive Productions (a division of sex toy retailer Good Vibrations). In independents you'll find everything from beautiful, black-and-white, shot-on-film features to white-knuckle, gritty S/M films shot in vivid color in actual dungeons. Most sex ed films come from independents.

In mainstream low-budget porn, which comprises the majority of what's available through your local retailers, the quality you are going to see is roughly that of regular (nonerotic) independent films, daytime soap operas, or daytime made-for-TV movies. These films feature simple sets, usually indoor filming in one location, standard lighting, digital cameras (which are what contribute to their "daytime TV" look and feel), and barely-present acting. Big-studio films can be surprisingly complex in script, have terrific cinematography, and show sexy, believable actors, though the movies (and actors) look purposely packaged and polished. Not surprisingly, the biggest studios have bigger budgets, access to better sets, actors who might have gone to acting school, writers with writing experience, and directors who are more likely to take their craft seriously. Some even use real film stock in their movies, which is costly but produces a higher-quality film, in look and feel. Sound quality is generally poor, even in the big-budget feature films. The independents can have the same quality range, but they are less likely to be found in a neighborhood video rental shop; they can be found more easily online or in a woman-oriented sex boutique (see Resources, Chapter 14, for recommendations).

As I'll detail later, not all porn has a plot, and in all-sex films you'll find that same variation in quality, from high-budget polish to low-budget rough edges. Many of these look like home movies, because that's what they are. The digital camera has made it possible for anyone with a little money and the right access to make and distribute a film. The medium to low-budget films will often contain extremely explicit ads for phone sex that are cheaply recycled footage from old films, with one hard-core come shot after another. Sometimes these ads are pretty aggressive, and contain scenes that might offend some people, such as "gaping anal" shots. Sometimes the immediacy of the ads' sexuality will make the films themselves seem anti-climactic; I know several women and men who get so hot so fast by the shocking ads at the beginning that they claim they "don't make it through" the ads, masturbating to orgasm before the ads are finished!

So, with rare exceptions, the video or DVD you bring home isn't going to be anything like the films you're used to watching at the local Cineplex. In terms of budget and therefore overall appearance, it'll be a close cousin of films you'd see on the Independent Film Channel, or B-movies. It's also important to keep in mind that you're going to be watching a film made to feature one thing: sex. Porn moviemakers think that the reason anyone (outside of their peers) is watching their film in the first place is to see hard-core, explicit sex. So the focus in each and every film will be the sex scenes, with everything else taking a back seat.

The need to focus on sex, combined with a small budget and minimal resources, often compromises vital aspects of the video's quality. Poor sound quality and "looped" scenes are an unfortunate result. Sound issues can mean hearing the sounds of the production crew, muffled or inaudible dialogue, or annoying background music—sometimes, incredibly enough, just music playing in the room where the actors are having sex. A huge complaint from viewers is having to sit through scenes that have been cut (often poorly) with looped film, meaning the action (such

• •

What the Hell Is a "Reverse Cowgirl"?

THE ADULT INDUSTRY might as well be its own country. It has its own strange customs—and its own language. Over the years, a lexicon has evolved out of slang, nicknames, and verbal shortcuts to comprise a whole world of terminology. Terms such as "wood," "reverse cowgirl," "DP," "pro-am," and "suitcase pimp" all describe specific body parts, positions, sex acts, film

subgenres, and the types of characters you'd find on or around a porn set. Just as the locals in a surf town have their own lingo, the porn industry takes the terms for granted and uses them as if everyone knew what they meant. You'll find them on box covers, in industry magazines, and in interviews with performers. Refer to the Glossary, Chapter 13, whenever you need a definition.

• •

as a close-up of a blow job) is edited in repetition to make the scene seem longer. Another annoying corner-cutter found on low-quality compilation and all-sex tapes is the technique of intermingling higher-quality scenes with badly filmed, lackluster scenes, for filler. You won't necessarily find these problems in the majority of tapes recommended in this book, but forewarned is forearmed, and if you watch adult videos you'll run into them eventually.

Formula Porn

This just in: Everything you see on TV and in movies is based on a tried-and-true formula—porn being no exception. When a Hollywood studio makes an "action" film, its head honchos know that audiences expect car chases, explosions, gunfire, plenty of fighting—and the hero rescuing a pretty girl (or vice versa) in the last shoot 'em up scene. Typically, though not always, genre films weave the story line around these formulaic expectations, often sacrificing character, setting, sound track, and film-making for plot. Genre films, like the classic spaghetti western, are often known for bad acting, predictable dialogue, and lack of story. You'll find the same limitations in much of mainstream porn—though these are the films I'll be steering you away from. In a typical adult video you will see six or seven sex scenes, including fellatio, cunnilingus, anal sex, a girl–girl scene, and lots of penis/vagina sex in doggie-style, missionary, cowgirl, and reverse cowgirl positions. The male ejaculation is almost always external, usually on the face (called a "facial"), and the sex is shown in extreme close-up. Sorry to ruin the ending for you.

Every mainstream porn film follows an unwritten rule to standardize the sex acts in a given film, and it's followed as strictly as a chemical formula to make bubble bath. This formula ensures that in each film there will be a standard set of sex acts (blow jobs, cunnilingus, vaginal and anal sex), positions (missionary, doggie style, reverse cowgirl) and couplings (male/female, two guys with one girl, two girls with one guy, girl–girl, and a group scene with four or more performers). Unless noted in the reviews, all films follow this formula.

Apart from the standard set of positions and couplings, most porn films feature actors and actresses who are polished and coiffed to fit the ideals of Southern California–style beauty, since that's where the majority of the industry is based. An oft-voiced complaint is that the men are acceptable even when unlovely in fitness and form, while the women's bodies must conform to a rigid standard of perfection: underweight, blonde hair, big lips, and big boobs (the plastic surgeons of Beverly Hills are always well represented). Without fail, the men always pull their penises out before orgasm and ejaculate so that the viewer can see it. To say the least, little emphasis is placed on female orgasm and ejaculation, but that's changing.

The Subgenres

In hard-core adult film, you'll find that all the films are grouped in general categories widely used by trade magazines, video retailers, and others in the industry. I've broken the categories down even further in the reviews to help you find what you're looking for in the store or at the Web retailer you're using. You might not find all these categories in your search, or you might find even more than what's listed here—again, there is no uniform method among retailers for labeling and stocking adult videos, and your searching might take you through some haphazard methods of categorization.

Bisexual

Bi videos are always in demand, and when they're hot, they're sizzling. However, generally budgets on bi films are low, and the sex is often lack-luster. It could be that the gay male actors are playing "bi for pay," that directors aren't drawn to the material, or simply that the low budgets aren't making anyone smile. You can find a few gems here and there, though, especially from independents cashing in on the high demand; I feature them in Chapter 10, "Lesbian, All-Girl, Bisexual, and Gay Features."

Classics

This term usually refers to famous or notorious films made in the 1970s or 1980s, such as *Deep Throat, Devil in Miss Jones,* and *Behind the Green*

Door, but can apply to any film from that time period. Many of these were shot on real film stock, so they look better and have a more cinematic feel, and have great actors, enthusiastic performances, and fantastic scripts. They're from a time gone by, so clothing, hairstyles, and body hair may seem dated. But the attention to plot, story, and sexual heat of these older films is astonishingly high, and it's worth giving them a try so that you can see what all the fuss was about—and view some really hot sex. See Chapter 7, "The Classics."

Educational

These videos have educational content but also feature explicit demonstrations or hard-core sex, or both. Many come from independents and can cover topics such as female ejaculation, male masturbation, learning S/M negotiation and techniques, or sex with someone with spinal-cord injury—to name just a few. Some companies have large catalogs and lengthy title lists, with several series tapes on particular subjects, such as sex and aging, or positions. Several porn stars have decided to show the world exactly how the pros do it, and their videos feature lessons on techniques, followed by demonstrations. Nina Hartley's many educational tapes showcase her training as a nurse as well as a porn actress and have excellent anatomical information. Many people like educational tapes because some show real couples having sex, often for the first time in front of a camera. See Chapter 11, "Educational Videos."

European

Porn from Europe is a much-loved thing, filmed in beautiful locations, with great visual film techniques, high budgets, and plenty of gorgeous European actors. Most European adult performers are very different in appearance from their "Silicone Valley" (read: surgically enhanced) counterparts, and their approach to sex is refreshingly open, playful, and unrushed. Often, the women exhibit their lusty sexuality in a way that comes across as more earthy and genuine than that of many American performers, while the men take the time to enjoy the women they're with. Unfortunately, sound quality is often poor, or the dialogue is badly dubbed (if at all). Some American directors travel to Europe to take advantage of the lovely locations and enthusiastic talent, and we all benefit when they do. European films are made in England, France, Italy, Czech Republic (principally in Prague), and Spain, but most of them are filmed in Budapest, Hungary, the European equivalent of Southern California's porn epicenter. Find selected European films in Chapter 6, "Feature Films," and many more in Chapter 8, "All Sex, No Plot."

Features

This large and unwieldy category includes all porn containing a plot, whether shot on film stock or on digital video (DV). You'll find incredible, full-length movies in this category, made by a whole roster of talented directors who are interesting and eccentric in the way they create movies. Each director has his or her own style. This is where you'll find erotic comedies, drama, crime films, love stories, and noir. Quite a few of these films are groomed for what the industry calls the couples market— ostensibly, pairs of men and women watching together. See Chapter 6, "Feature Films."

Gay Male

The vast world of gay male porn has a whole set of its own subgenres, such as all-sex, plot-driven, bears (big hairy men), twinks (young-looking waifs), European (usually Eastern European), gay and bi (gay men with a woman thrown in the middle), S/M, military, locker-room fetish, interracial, and more. See Chapter 10, "Lesbian, All-Girl, Bisexual, and Gay Features."

Gonzo

In 1989 a new genre was born: *gonzo,* films with no plot in which the man with the camera also directs the action, occasionally getting involved and giving the viewer a first-person experience. Taking its name from writer Hunter S. Thompson's irreverent, improvised situational style of journalism, the genre gave every camcorder owner the feeling he or she could make porn, and made voyeurism into a style of video production.

Ed Powers and John Stagliano (aka Buttman) pioneered gonzo and are considered by many to be at the top of the form, though they have heavy competition from filmmakers such as Adam Glasser (Seymore Butts) and Ben Dover. See also, "Pro-Am" and "Wall-to-Wall." Find gonzo videos in Chapter 8, "All Sex, No Plot."

Hentai, sometimes called Anime

Although seldom found in the adult section of your local video store or in the adult-only stores, adults-only animated Japanese videos can be found in many video stores specializing in cult and foreign films. *Hentai* videos are cartoons for adults, and contain explicit sex in every imaginable taboo situation. Illustrated in a classic Japanese style, the action is colorful and exaggerated, the characters have huge eyes and tiny mouths, and the flow of animation is stylistically choppy. Many fans of the genre love the fantastic sexual situations, which often include sex with monsters, supernatural beings, and alien animals. It's not uncommon for these films to depict sibling sex and incest taboos. Transsexual themes are also common. The animated nature of the genre allows for full fantasy exploration (especially the physically impossible), and gives free reign for some Western taboos to be interpreted differently in Japanese culture. For instance, the women often look like underage schoolgirls, but it should be noted that women who attend college in Japan must wear the same regulation uniforms as the young girls, and the lack of pubic hair is the result of a Japanese taboo about depicting pubic hair. Although it recently became legal to show pubic hair, many animators still choose not to show any, to comply with community standards. If you're interested in exploring *Hentai*, start with Gilles Poitras's book, *Anime Essentials: Every Thing a Fan Needs to Know.*

Independent

These are films released by independent distribution sources and small production companies. These films will yield the most diverse selection of casts, sex acts, and points of view. Many educational films come from independents, and you'll also find everything in this category from film-festival award-winning lesbian movies shot on film to rough, gritty S/M videos shot in San Francisco dungeons. What distinguishes an independent production company is that it makes and distributes the films itself, outside the major porn companies and distribution channels, giving it more creative and artistic freedom. No one is telling it what to do, or how it has to make its product profitable, and many of the resulting film projects are both outstanding and arousing.

Lesbian, Girl–Girl, or All-Girl

Guess what? The women in mainstream porn who are in videos with "lesbian" in the title are rarely lesbians. Surprised? I hope not. They're porn stars who "work with women," though sometimes they're bisexual in real life, and occasionally they're really lesbians. That's why "girl–girl" and "all-girl" are more appropriate words for their titles, and when you see a real lesbian film vs. a girl–girl video, you'll see the difference right away. Plenty of terrific all-girl series exist on the market, in videos like the *No Man's Land* series, featuring porn actresses who clearly enjoy their work. But very few mainstream "lesbian" porn films include the whole spectrum of thriving lesbian sexuality. When you get your hands on a genuine, lesbian-made video, you'll see how intense and incredible this expression of sexuality is. And the real lesbian films are quite popular, with more and more coming on the market each year. You'll find them among features, all-sex, S/M, and other subgenres.

Pro-Am

Short for "professional amateur," pro-am films involve participants who are new to adult film or who may be having sex with professionals for the first time. The genre also includes solo women in their first experience on camera. The videos are all-sex, often with a loose theme, and the quality varies widely. You'll come across tapes with hot newcomers having amazing sex, as well as people who are obviously not newcomers at all (having great sex, too). You'll also find bored and boring actors, or experienced "newcomers" faking it badly. See also, "Gonzo" and "Wall-to-Wall."

S/M

Videos in this genre include those featuring B/D (bondage and discipline), S/M (sadomasochism), or D/S (dominance and submission). Specialties range from spanking, whipping, caning, and restraint with ropes and leather, to erotic torture (with everything from clothespins to mild electricity), "forced" submission, and slave training. Some are set in professional dungeons, and all activities take place between consenting adults who have negotiated the scene beforehand. Some tapes will say "S/M" or "in leather" on the box cover, but in fact only have scenes of actors in S/M gear holding a whip while they have sex. You will almost never see a tape that combines both S/M and sex on one tape. Quality ranges from lush and beautiful to low budget and rough. Why don't they show S/M with sex? Read why in "S/M Features," Chapter 9.

• •

How Many Categories Can There Possibly Be?

RETAILERS AND WEBSITES want to direct customers to their chosen category of adult video as fast as possible, but the result is a million crazy classifications, from "straight" all the way down to "hairy all-girl underwater naked midget battles to the death." Okay, I made that one up, but you get the idea. And yes, many of the categories will shock and offend, confuse or arouse, and promise the impossible.

Here is a sample from the website www.talkingblue.com: Adult Mainstream, Amateur Sex, Anal Queens, Animation, Asian Sex, Big Boob Babes, Black Erotica, Body Builders, Cat Fighting, Classics on Film, Compilations, Couples, Deep Throating, Double Penetration, Español, Euro, Facials, Fat Femme Fatales, Freaky Sex, Gang Bangers, Gonzo, Hairy Humpers, Incest, Interracial, Itty Bitty Titties, Latin Lovers, Leather and Lace, Lesbians, Lingerie, Mature, Midget Movies, Oral, Orgy, Parodies, Satanic Erotica, Sex Education, Shaving, Solo, Strap-on Babes, Strippers, Swingers, Tasteful Toes, Threesome, Vintage Voyeurism, Weird Sex, Wet and Messy, White House Sex.

• •

"Specialty"

When porn is labeled *specialty,* it usually depicts a sex act or interest that falls outside conventional heterosexual tastes—and might cover ground that some find shocking. This industry-labeled category includes *bukkake,* transsexuals, fat folks, elderly (sometimes geriatric), fetishes (such as foot, breast, panties, lactation, pregnant women, hairy women), and more. For some readers this may seem like a bizarre cabinet of sexual curiosities, but for others with far-out tastes it provides a safe place where they can find what they want. Thrown into the "specialty" category is the recently emerged category of extreme porn: videos that combine sex with themes or activities that are intended to shock or disgust the viewer.

Wall-to-Wall

These videos are all-sex, no plot—usually tapes of sex scenes strung together loosely by a theme (like amateurs) or focusing on a sex act (such as fellatio), or both, as in first-time anal sex. These seldom are shot on film or have high production values, but some, such as John Leslie's *Voyeur* series, have both qualities. The sex in this subgenre can be boring, but often it's incendiary, as even the low-budget guys with the handicams can capture incredible, raw, unscripted sex in scenes that can never be repeated. Quality varies widely, and you'll find a lot of series tapes here, which take a theme and run with it for sometimes as many as forty installments. Also overlaps into the categories "Gonzo," "All-Girl," and "Pro-Am."

Woman-Directed

Going where no woman has gone before? Maybe not, but in the past decade, women have stepped up to the clapper board and started directing their own films. Tired of the same old points of view and driven by their own creative fires, many former adult actresses decided to try out the view from the other side of the camera lens, and found that they like it there—and do fine work. The success of their films has made many of these women power-players in the industry, and for good reason. Their films are well-shot, high-quality, complete films, with lots of attention paid to female pleasure. Veronica Hart, Chloe, and Candida Royalle, for example, make fantastic, story-driven features, while other women like Shane show us that not all women want a plot and that the gals can be just like the guys in making hot and nasty, women-oriented, all-sex videos.

5

Common Concerns About Content

I walked in the room, and there were these hideous close-ups of a vagina on TV—it made me afraid to let my boyfriends go down on me for many years.

Everyone has concerns about porn. And many people run up against these concerns when they want to investigate adult videos—they are stopped, or their arousal is derailed by their concerns about content. Some people will put in a tape, see something that offends or upsets them, hit the "eject" button, and never experiment with porn again. While it's true that everyone has concerns, and that there is probably something out there to offend everyone, most people don't know that their concerns can help them select the right tape, and that the viewing choices in porn are many.

Avoiding What You Don't Like

You can avoid seeing sexual images or activities that you don't want to see, though some things, like facial ejaculation and anal sex, are practically in every video. It will help to be aware of your own expectations. This will help you make a selection that won't leave you high and dry or, in the worst-case scenario, angry or disgusted.

Knowing what you like and dislike can help enormously when selecting a tape. You can single out many of your preferences before you rent or buy, and then skip the parts you don't care for. The reviews on independent porn websites like Blue Door and on women-owned sex toy websites (and in catalogs) are very helpful in these matters—I should know, I've been writing these reviews at women-owned adult retailer Good Vibrations for five years. The reviews and ratings can also help you select videos that will help you find things you don't usually see on the blue screen, such as an all-natural cast (that is, actresses without breast implants), internal ejaculation, attention to cinematography and lighting, great acting, and excellent plot.

As a general rule, most women-owned sex toy stores never carry films that are demeaning or abusive toward women or that contain racist or discriminatory content—of any kind. They often have complicated screening procedures that make sure their tapes portray healthy sexuality, meaning that the videos depict positive attitudes about sex (no sexual shame allowed!), and show women getting off as much as the men. Such videos always pay attention to female pleasure. The porn these shops carry won't model unsafe sex practices, such as inserting anything anally that can get "lost" in the rectum. Whenever something borderline or potentially button-pressing comes up in a tape with an overwhelming redeeming quality, such as a stand-out sex scene or underrepresented content, they often make sure that their product descriptions warn customers about it.

Frankly, certain things in porn are going to be hard to avoid. Facial ejaculation (men ejaculating on women's faces) is pretty much a standard. So are boob jobs. I hear a lot of complaints about both of these things, yet some porn viewers enjoy watching "facials," or seeing women with large breasts, authenticity notwithstanding. But if you want to avoid facials, look for porn made by feminist-identified women directors like Candida Royalle. Finding videos with all-natural starlets is a little trickier, but more of them are in the business now than were five years ago.

Porn's Maladies

Porn is a fantasy world, but whose fantasy world *is* it? On the one hand porn films appear to be made for a narrowly defined audience of single heterosexual men all of whom like to see big-boobed blondes engaged in predictable sex acts. On the other hand, it looks like the makers of porn are trying to appeal to as many viewers as possible, with a resulting mish-mash of sexual activities.

Usually, for one reason or another, everyone has a complaint about porn. Many people feel that their sexuality isn't being reflected on the flickering screen. They're right—porn does not represent the sexual diversity we encounter in real life. Is porn sexist? Yes. Is porn racist? Yes. Porn isn't created for you, or for me—it's for that fantasy audience the producers and distributors *think* is watching porn. And most porn producers and distributors believe the audience is all white, all male, unintelligent, desperate for any kind of sexual imagery, lonely, insecure about their penis size, and possessing unrefined sexual tastes.

They're wrong. The fact is, we're the ones watching. And we're not just "raincoaters"—far from it, in fact. Porn is for those of us who like sex, like movies, and enjoy watching other people get off, and we're a lot more sexually sophisticated than some people think. And some of us like some of the things we see, others dislike certain things, and some of us could care less about the details. So what bothers you?

I'm afraid it will upset me.

It's unsettling to feel aroused by images we find offensive on one level or another. If you're ashamed of sex, you're likely to feel embarrassed by the explicit imagery in porn. Embarrassment manifests in several guises: shame, anger, depression, self-hatred—plus arousal. If you find the image of a woman being graphically penetrated upsetting, yet simultaneously arousing, you will likely feel alarmed by your own feelings. But for most people, watching women have sex is incredibly arousing, not upsetting or degrading. Some experience the seemingly contradictory feelings of upset and arousal, and find that it enhances their experience. Those comfortable with their sexuality and personal boundaries may enjoy "visiting" the experience of upset/arousal much like a roller coaster ride, or a scary movie. The best way to understand your reaction to porn, female sexuality, and your own sexuality is to examine your feelings. Are you ashamed of your own body, fantasies, or desires? Think about what you really want: hot sex in a healthy relationship, comfort about your own sexuality, or making your sex life more fun and adventurous. Make your goal a great sex life—in whatever definition you prefer and whatever style you feel comfortable—instead of feeling bad or worried.

Porn is in the eye of the beholder. It's degrading to you if you're degraded by it. Situations where people are behaving offensively onscreen can make anyone feel pretty bad, but on a personal level, you can call the shots about who or what makes you more (or less) of a person.

The women have obviously fake breasts.

This is a big complaint among both female and male viewers. And porn *is* a heavily augmented industry, right up there with professional dancing and modeling and Hollywood acting. The business of the body, the image, requires focus on the performer as product, and many women (and men) mold themselves to standards of conformity or what they read as popular desire in their quest for success—and in both Hollywood and porn, surgical augmentation has been the norm. In Hollywood as in the porn industry, the average for augmentation procedures, such as liposuction, is every six months.

I'll argue that physical beauty is open to interpretation—what's hot for you is a turn-off for someone else. Some people who watch explicit films get turned on by large-breasted women, and our mass culture feeds the stereotyping of big breasts equaling sexiness. Adult actresses and strippers find across the board that when they get their boobs done, lo and behold, they make more money. The problem is that you can usually tell when those breasts are fake, and a lot of people find them, well, kinda creepy. You can often see incision scars around the nipples, under the breast, adjacent to the armpit, or on the side. Implants make the breasts sit up quite high and move in a way that looks very different from natural breasts (if they move much at all). When the actress leans over they often look lumpy. And the very presence of evident implants can remind the viewer of surgery—not very arousing.

Not all porn actresses have surgery, though, and there are lots of hot all-natural gals out there. But some get a series of surgeries, and a few have unusual procedures performed. Some porn actresses have had cosmetic surgery on their labia and clitoris to make their genitals look more lean, and I know of at least one actress who had cheek implants so that her face would look more sculpted when she gave blow jobs. Surgical augmentation became very popular in porn in the late 1980s, turned into an adult industry standard in the 1990s, and is now becoming less of a standard as the adult industry finds its market expanding to a more opinionated, more critical viewership.

It's not easy, but you can narrow down your viewing choices to watching films that feature all-natural women. There's more porn for this preference appearing on the market every day. Entire series cater to viewers who prefer natural women, and some big-breasted series even employ only naturally endowed women. Certain films and series don't market the women as "all-naturals" but will use them exclusively anyway. And you can almost always find all-natural women in independent porn and instructional videos. Use the "fast forward" button judiciously to find the actresses who turn you on for whatever reason, and don't be shy about acknowledging those reasons. Also, learn the names of stars whose physical endowments—surgically enhanced or not—turn you on, and avoid the ones you don't want to see.

The men aren't to my liking, and the same ones are in all the films.

This is an industry that chooses women for their attractiveness, the men for their "wood" (ability to get and keep an erection). Being a man in porn is not as easy as many think—it's not that you "get to have sex with hot chicks all day long." You have to have an overly large penis; be able to get it up on command in front of a cast, crew, and camera; and then keep it up until someone else says you're done, which could be a very long time. At that point you have to orgasm on command, in front of everyone, probably in a difficult position—and it's best if your load is large and shoots far. And, hopefully, you should be somewhat pleasant to work with. Because, after all, it is a job.

That's one reason you won't usually find "hunks" in porn—unless it's gay male porn. Gay men's porn is all about the hot studly men, and features a more diverse selection of body types, all of whom are coincidentally hung like horses. The guys in gay male porn will range from tan, coiffed, and more muscular than your average guy—beefy but "clean-looking"—to sexy older men, waifish young things, and tough guys of every color. Many straight women enjoy watching gay male porn because of the way that the male body is eroticized and shown in all its sexual variety.

Straight porn lacks hunks for another reason. It may be hearsay but is a widely held belief: Lots of folks think that the men in straight porn are purposely selected to be less attractive than your average guy. The belief is that hot hunks will intimidate the male viewer, and that watching a good-looking star with the fantasy woman onscreen would bruise his ego. This way, the male viewer's ego stays intact.

Well, besides the unusual physical qualifications of the male porn star, the other fact remains that many of the men in porn have gotten onscreen by being in the right place at the right time—with an easily controlled erection. There are lots of attractive men coming into the business these days. If you don't find a male star that appeals to you, keep looking, and check out different genres and eras. Some porn has no men at all, and some feature men only as props. For instance, in many Andrew Blake films you often won't even see the male actors' heads or faces, just their lower bodies!

I don't like anal sex/oral sex/lesbian scenes/facial come shots....

It's difficult to avoid these popular sex acts in porn. While anal sex with women as the recipient was rarely seen in the heterosexual films of the

1970s and 1980s, by the 1990s it had become a standard. A few tapes here and there have no anal; for example, very few of director Candida Royalle's films have anal sex in them. But usually anal, oral, and girl–girl scenes are part and parcel of the porn formula. Look closely at the film reviews throughout the book—I'll indicate which films omit these activities.

The men only come on the outside of the women, and the women never come at all.

External ejaculation is another of porn's standard practices, one nearly impossible to avoid. A few films here and there contain scenes where the man comes inside the woman, and they're rare enough to warrant a mention in the review sections. The practice of men pulling out to come has been around as long as porn. This is done so that the audience can see the orgasm, the peak and release of the sex act. It's the proof the guy came. Until recently, from the medical community to the adult community, little value was placed on female orgasm, and so male orgasm was—and still is—the centerpiece. Most heterosexual men love to see a woman getting off, but the makers of porn have been slow to focus on authentic female orgasms. More and more films are coming out that focus on female pleasure, and on the women getting off—for real.

Only in the past ten years have shots of facial ejaculation, or "facials," become commonplace in porn. Some people find this degrading or disgusting, while others—including female viewers—find it highly arousing. Still others couldn't care less where the guy comes as long as they can see it. Some people think facials are boring and predictable, and would rather see the come shot on another body part they prefer, like the woman's breasts. If you dislike facials, look for porn aimed at the couples' market or from independent filmmakers such as Libido Films.

How do they do it with those fingernails?

Good question. Many female porn stars have fingernails that look like talons from a bird of prey, and quite a few women see the stars fingering themselves on screen and wince. Those fingernails look like they'd be difficult to rub a clit with—and they definitely don't look safe for insertion. As with everything in porn, use the "fast forward" button without hesitation if fake nails bother you, but also know that those porn star nails are not the glue-on kind. They're acrylic, made part of the actual fingernail, and won't come off to stay lodged in any body cavity. And usually they're not as sharp as they look but quite rounded at the tips. Also, these women are pros, and have had a lot of practice not scratching themselves or their partners.

The performers look like they're "going through the motions."

Then turn off the tape and get another one. You don't have to settle for mediocre porn with uninterested actors. Unfortunately, because these films are made on limited budgets and porn performers need to make lots of movies to earn a living, many bored-looking people end up in videos around the world. Not all videos are like that, however, and oodles of movies show people who really can't keep their hands off each other. Porn with chemistry that sizzles sells well, and pornographers are waking up to this fact, being motivated to feature more, and more honestly hot, scenes in their films.

Women directors are a great place to start, and you'll find lots of heat in independent films, as well as instructional tapes. Entire series show real couples really doing it, and "amateur" porn with its unscripted nature as well as European films all pack genuine heat. While many mainstream porn directors have great films but cold sex scenes, a few directors (John Leslie being one) shoot scenes that could burn a hole through your screen. Some mainstream porn films even have real-life couples. The *Deep Inside* series focuses on an actress's favorite scenes—and you can see why these are favorites, some even showcasing a scene where the actress has sex with someone she loves.

The music is lame.

Yes, it is. Bad music ruins a good sex scene, and in fact music in general, if it's not to your taste, can be too distracting. Many of the all-sex, no-plot directors don't use music of any kind, featuring the natural sounds of the actors having sex (Christoph Clark is a great example). Unfortunately, some will try to dress up a video or correct spoiled sound with music that is *their* idea of sexy—usually not yours. If you get a video with irritating music but great visuals, turn the sound down, or off. Play your own music if you want.

The genital close-ups are more medical than sexual.

Close-ups are the industry standard. With the exception of independent adult films and porn directed by certain women, you're going to be watching giant, floating, seemingly dismembered and brightly lit penises going into vaginas, mouths, and asses on your TV screen. No mystery, no question about what's going on here—and that's part of the reason you'll see it. It might feel more like a documentary than a sexy movie, but these shots are the bread and butter of the videos. The close-ups present the sex right there, in your face, without the distraction of the actors to take your attention away from one thing—the onscreen sex and its direct rela-tionship to your masturbation. While close-ups are a little much for some people, seeing sexual anatomy in motion is an expectation that many viewers have when getting a tape for masturbation purposes. Still, I'll agree that it's boring when that's all you get, with nothing else to tweak the imagination. If you don't want to see any close-ups, you can watch soft-core versions, independent films labeled "no genital close-ups," or films by a number of female directors.

Don't the performers know it's not safe to have unprotected sex?

In porn's intent to portray harmless fantasy, it often gives us a fantasy world that can only ever be that: pure fantasy. Every thinking person who watches porn makes a silent agreement when he or she pops the tape in. While on a good day porn delivers the fantasies well, in the realm of portraying healthy and safe sex it will always fail. The main reason is that pornographers want to give viewers the fantasy sex they demand. Fantasy sex doesn't require condoms, doesn't allow for the possibility that hepatitis will be transmitted by toys that have been inserted anally, and doesn't worry its pretty little head about the many dangers of unprotected sex with multiple partners or strangers. Instead, we get our fantasies, *and* a huge misrepresentation of how to stay alive and actively sexual in today's world.

True, some porn stars have been diagnosed with STDs—including AIDS—while working in the business (and "working in the business" means having sex with other actors). The most famous case was legendary über-dick John Holmes, who made films and had unprotected sex with actresses on-camera after testing positive for HIV. Holmes did not inform his coworkers, and put many people's lives at risk. In the late 1990s, Marc Wallice contracted HIV and continued working, infecting four of his female costars. Call it ignorant or call it murderous, their actions sent a wake-up call to everyone who works in porn.

HIV isn't the only thing you can get from unprotected sex. Herpes, syphilis, genital warts, gonorrhea, chlamydia, bacterial infections, and other diseases and viruses can be passed by one single encounter sans condom. Former adult actress Sharon Mitchell saw the risks far outweighing the benefits of working in adult films, and responded by founding AIM, the Adult Industry Medical Healthcare Foundation. In 1998 the adult entertainment industry suffered an HIV outbreak involving many people that Mitchell knew when she was in movies. The industry gave her the support that she needed to found AIM, a nonprofit organization serving sex workers and the general public in areas of HIV testing, STD testing, GYN services and treatment, counseling of many types, and sponsoring industry-related educational groups as resources for informational materials.

AIM's motto is "Health for the sex worker in body, mind, emotion and spirit!" In a recent collection of data, AIM administered voluntary tests to a group consisting primarily of adult film workers. Of 483 people tested between October 2001 and March 2002, about 40 percent had at least one STD. None of the tests came up positive for HIV, Mitchell said. The 40 percent infection rate compares to that of the mainstream (nonadult industry) population: according to San Francisco Sex Information, around 40 percent of the nonporn population has some form of sexually transmitted condition, too.

• •

A Reviewer's Complaints

AFTER YEARS OF WATCHING PORN on a daily basis for my job—as well as my personal pleasure!—I have my own list of complaints. Cookie-cutter performers and safe-sex questions aside, my axes to grind are critiques of technical flaws than could be easily overcome:

• Looped and recycled footage to extend scenes

• Phone sex commercials seemingly from the 1980s

• Embarrassing grammar and spelling mistakes on box covers

• Camera flashbulbs during sex scenes (for boxcover stills)

• Hearing the director or technician when you shouldn't

• Box cover lies about content and production values

• Bad special effects

• Low VHS tape quality

• Low DVD quality and poor DVD menus

• •

AIM Healthcare serves more than 400 clients a month and is expanding into a larger, full-service organization. Since its inception, it has successfully lowered the spread of HIV in porn, and has certainly increased awareness among performers. By adult industry standards, an adult entertainment worker should be tested for HIV/AIDS every thirty days, and though much of the industry supports mandatory monthly testing for chlamydia and gonorrhea, there is no standard for testing for other STDs. Most—though not all—producers/directors will not hire an actor if he or she lacks an HIV test less than 30 days old, while testing for other STDs is on a case-by-case basis depending on performers and directors. Most gang-bang shoots require the participants to arrive with certification from AIM that they have tested negative for both HIV and other STDs. However, since the industry is self-regulating in all aspects of testing and condom use, safer-sex risk assessment ultimately falls into the hands of the performers.

AIM uses an HIV test that produces results in one to three business days, and it is one of the most reliable tests for HIV. AIM uses the costly and highly effective PCRDNA test because it is the best test for quick-result, early detection of HIV and also functions as a monitoring screening test for adult entertainment workers and the sexually active. The standard test for HIV is the ELISA test, which has a window period of up to six months because it tests only for the antibody to HIV, not for the virus. The PCRDNA test looks for the virus itself and can detect HIV after about two weeks (give or take a day or two). So far, AIM has reported only two false positives and no false negatives. They confirm each positive result with further standard HIV tests like ELISA.

But these precautions are not foolproof, especially with the variety and number of unsafe practices engaged in by porn performers, including ejaculations in the eyes and unsafe anal insertions. Read more about what's really safe and what isn't in Chapter 12, "Safer Sex in Porn."

Does Porn Degrade Women?

For most people, the idea of a woman being degraded, shamed, or violated for someone else's viewing pleasure just isn't arousing. A number of people have strong convictions about pornography and women; some of these folks believe that graphic erotic images of women are harmful, regardless of either the participation level of the woman in the image or the intent of the viewer. Another perspective sees adult film as an industry that forces women into humiliation. After all, no woman in her right mind would do something like that. Not for pleasure. Or would she?

Those who believe in porn's alleged degradation of women are making a lot of assumptions about the people in porn, specifically the women, and about the people viewing the imagery:

- The woman is ashamed of what she is doing—or should be.
- She isn't enjoying it, or women as a class can't and don't enjoy certain types of sex.
- She is sexually receptive and therefore less than human.
- The viewer is always male.
- The actress doesn't know the effect her image has—that porn leads to real-life acts of rape and degradation.
- Open sexual desire is shameful for all participants, on- and offscreen.

How can anyone possibly know how every viewer or participant feels, or sees themself? The answer is that no one can. Each individual must be allowed to decide what is healthy and okay for them—no one else can decide that for you, or for another person.

Questions of Age and Consent

The women in porn participate on every level, from actresses who do it proudly for the money and those who have their hottest, most orgasmic sex while being filmed, to actresses who do something they feel bad about but do it nevertheless. However, the women who feel bad about it are in the minority and don't stick around long. It's just like every other job—some have a passion for the work, others see it as an enjoyable moneymaking activity, while some have mixed feelings about how they're making a buck, and for still others porn is just a job. Some women can get off on living out their sexual fantasies: letting themselves be watched, being the center of affection and attention, getting sexual with other women, getting sexual with a stranger, trying new fantasies in erotic role-play scenarios, and, yes, acting out "being used" or "degraded." Make no mistake, there is never a point when the actresses are not doing what they want to be doing; they can walk off the set at any time. To get a fresh perspective on this, explore the writings (and films) from women who have enriched their sexual, political, and spiritual lives working in adult films, such as Annie Sprinkle's *Post Porn Modernist* and Carol Queen's *Real Live Nude Girl*.

A lot of women and men want to be in porn. It's lucrative, it's exciting—but it's also hard work and a tough field to be successful in. To be cast in an adult video, the performers have to want to be (and must prove that they will be) a reliable and interesting performer—otherwise, pornographers will pass them by, moving on to the next exciting new prospective "talent." But once a performer finds a director or producer who says "okay, you're hired," the performer must provide a valid ID (with the performer's real name and age) and sign a release. The ID and information is collected prior to the shoot, then kept on file at a location that is given

Traci Lords

BORN AND RAISED in Ohio in 1968, Traci Lords ran away to Southern California at age 15. Armed with a fake ID, she jumped into adult film and quickly made a name for herself as the most vociferous and sexually wild vixen in porn circa 1984. With both the industry and viewers unaware of her age, Lords made films for two years. While her autobiography, *Traci Lords: Underneath it All*, claims she made 20 films, the Internet Movie Database and Internet Adult Film Database credit her with over 100 films. Her sexual appetite brought to his knees every man she came across, but she brought the whole adult indus-

try to its knees when the secret of her age was revealed just after her eighteenth birthday. The industry scrambled to recall every Lords film ever made for fear of federal prosecution, and the feds had already started procedures when the case suddenly had to be dropped— Traci had used her fake ID to get a U.S. passport, fooling the federal government as well. The industry was mad as hell at Traci, and she was effectively blacklisted from adult—though this notoriety helped fuel her success in TV and "mainstream" film (with much thanks to cult director John Waters for casting her in *Cry Baby*).

on both the box cover of the film as well as in the credits of the film itself. The address is clearly visible, with the time, title, and date of production.

The Women

All kinds of women are attracted to working in porn; they come from all walks of life, and in all shapes and sizes. The majority of women you'll see in porn, however, tend to fit pretty narrow stereotypes of conventional female beauty—though, as you will see in the films described in this book, this is not the rule. The women and men in porn get their jobs because they do one thing in particular very, very well: they have incredible, hot sex while the camera rolls—and while you watch. These women like sex, like to be watched while they do it, and enjoy showing their enthusiasm and lust. Both male and female performers emit a sensuality that you don't see every day, and the best of the breed love to crank it up onscreen. Their sexual heat is undeniable, and their uncontrollable hunger for each other can be an instant turn-on. Great porn performers know that it's their job to turn you, the viewer, on—and they clearly enjoy their work.

Porn performers are selected for their gigs based on appearance, willingness to perform, and physical skills. They keep their jobs and become successful if they are reliable and relatively easy to work with, have a "glow" or magnetism, are above average in conventional standards of attractiveness, or can act (though not always a requirement for all sex features), and they shine with passion for their on-camera sex partners. Porn folks, like their Hollywood counterparts, are very regular-looking people, just packaged very, very well with lots of makeup, professional hair styling, body waxing, lighting (and airbrushing, if stills), and many having had some type of surgical augmentation.

The porn industry has filmed hundreds of male and literally thousands of female performers. Many will work for a few years, and then switch occupations, making keeping track of them impossible. Some get out to make better money elsewhere, because they find the work distasteful, or because it's tough to hack it in an industry that is hard on your body and psyche and is irritatingly obsessed with youth. But those who do stick around are star-quality, and amazing to watch at work. Newcomers are thrilling, and experienced players emit a focused heat onscreen.

Most women in adult start out as strippers, or erotic dancers in clubs. Several will work a nationwide circuit of clubs, and make the move to porn slowly, or all at once if their first few films are successful. The really lucky women will rise to the top, winning awards for performances, becoming "contract girls," or grabbing the reins and writing and directing their own porn. Most women in porn also work the nationwide strip circuit for their entire careers as a lucrative adjunct to their film work.

Contract girls are women who are such hot tickets that a big production company, such as VCA or Vivid, will sign them to exclusive contracts.

Ginger Lynn: The First Contract Girl

BEFORE THE TRACI LORDS SCANDAL, when Lords was a phenomenon to contend with, a new company, Vivid Video, tried to mastermind a gimmick that could compete and land it on the map—thus conceiving the "contract girl." Wanting to focus on a single actress and have its first feature titled with her name to tie in their company and marketing campaign, Vivid chose the other top star in the business, Ginger Lynn, for the first contract girl. Vivid did a whole series with Lynn that was extremely successful, prompting more contract girls, and watching other companies imitate the contract girl marketing, packaging, and promotion of their top stars. Contract girls are chosen from new or reigning superstars, and go under contract for a length of time or number of titles—but a year is average. Big-studio Metro signs up different starlets to fit different niches; some do gonzos, some do features.

Like many adult film stars, Ginger Lynn came to California in the early 1980s with her sights set on film stardom, hoping to make it big—and in fact reigned as the biggest star in porn from 1985 through 1987. She starred in hundreds of films, most notably the Mitchell Brothers' *The Grafenberg Spot* and Gregory Dark's *New Wave Hookers*.

Lynn went on to break into mainstream films and television, where her talent and beauty have brought her a measure of success under her real name, Ginger Lynn Allen. She made news in 1992 when her relationship with actor Charlie Sheen hit the tabloids. Lynn is currently a VCA contract star, and has set the screen on fire with her stellar acting skills in films such as *Torn, Taken,* and *White Lightning*.

These women are respected and well paid, and though they can only work for one company they have a lot more say in the projects they're involved in than other performers. Often, outside of major companies, the women and men have no say in whom they work with or what project they're working on—it's a job like any other.

Women directors are an exciting breed of porn performer. Until lately, they've been women who put in a fair amount of time in front of the camera, working through porn's classic eras (1970s and 1980s) to now write, direct, and produce their own films. Recently, other young performers (such as Shane and Chloe) have chosen to do the same, and all around the results are incredible. Former and present female stars bring something to making porn that you just can't find in regular porn—especially the focus on female pleasure, attention to production values, and authentic female orgasms. Read about the many diverse women making mainstream porn in Chapter 6, "Feature Films," and Chapter 8, "All Sex, No Plot."

Feature Films

*I guess I'm old fashioned—but I like a film with
well-developed characters and a plot that grabs my
attention. What can I say? I'm spoiled by Hollywood.
I didn't even watch porn until I discovered Paul
Thomas—especially Bobby Sox. Could it be that I
identify with a washed-up, alcoholic filmmaker trying
to get it on with teenaged girls? Hmmm…*

Porn with a plot is considered a feature film—that is, a movie
with story, characters, and all the qualities of a regular film—
but with the good parts left in. Instead of fading out after the
first kiss, or panning the camera away when the sex starts, or
showing the couple waking up the next morning, the camera stays right there, so you see every arousing detail.
Features have flavor and style, can communicate interesting
ideas, and get you involved with the story so you can

become excited on many levels. A good feature will pull you in, involve you, turn you on, and push you over the orgasmic edge—and be worthy of a rewind. Each feature is unique to the script, actors, budget, and director, though each director has their own style of filming a story, and filming sex.

Features are released both by big studios and by independent artists. Big studios, such as VCA, Vivid, Wicked, and Metro, will have high-budget, polished feature films that use porn stars and employ the standard formula for sex scenes. They contract with in-house directors, who each have their own style. In choosing a good feature film, what matters is not who the studios are, but rather which directors make the films *you* like. By contrast, independents make films on small budgets, cast actors who look more like everyday people (or use nonactor amateurs in acting roles), and often (but not always) present unformulaic sex. Independent porn exists outside mainstream porn, just like Hollywood—except as of yet there's no Sundance Film Festival of independent porn, though some of the films do occasionally make their way through Sundance and other big festivals. And for the most part, as with Hollywood's awards shows, inde-pendents are seldom recognized at mainstream award events.

One of the best ways to find an adult film style you like is to search for videos by director. Certain feature directors take themselves seriously as filmmakers, and create films for an audience they believe to be con-noisseurs of both porn and film. Some directors make great films that parody adult filmmaking or the adult industry experience—intended for an industry-savvy audience. A few feature directors are simply trying to make a buck, creating porn with a plot for a variety of reasons, usually because their producer wants porn for the "couples market"—soft-focus, romantic tales created for what they perceive to be a gentler, female audi-ence. Feature directors are both male and female, with style and intention all over the spectrum.

Adult Feature Directors

Some people love David Lynch films, while others would rather drop a hammer on their toe than watch *Blue Velvet*. John Waters has a huge cult following and adoring fans, while at the same time some people can't believe that anyone watches his films. Many people enjoy the fantasy-based, feel-good movies of Steven Spielberg and George Lucas, yet others retch at the thought that viewers fork over millions of dollars to watch them. Ridley Scott movies aren't for everyone, nor are Stanley Kubrick's, and, come to think of it, just as many viewers are split over directors such as Peter Jackson, Mel Brooks, Werner Herzog, Robert Altman, Roman Polanski, Martin Scorsese, and Quentin Tarantino. The mark of a director on a film is as unique and indelible as a thumbprint. Granted, you won't find the caliber or technical expertise of these big-studio names in adult film, but you *will* find that who directs the film you watch makes all the difference in the world.

Hollywood and the porn industry have much in common, from studio systems and starlets to in-house directors and independent mavericks. Filmmaking as a whole is a vast universe, but finding the porn you like is really much like finding any movie you'd like to watch, and understanding how each filmmaker's vision is focused through the lens of that individual creator. Each director has their own style, which makes all the difference in the finished film. However, unlike Hollywood, where most films are essentially made by consensus and seldom have the stamp of an individual voice, porn is almost always an expression of the director, overlaid by the flavor or theme of the production company. Porn has a lot more room for creativity than do mass-marketed nonerotic films—it only lacks Hollywood's outrageous budgets.

Directors and series producers differ greatly with respect to how they believe sex should be portrayed, and have widely ranging views on a definition of "hot sex." In many ways this is a boon for us viewers, as we are a highly diverse audience of porn consumers. Because porn is the one thing in the world that as a whole shows sexuality in most every permutation, we stand a chance of finding the very thing that we're looking for. But in many cases, the filmmakers disagree with one another on how it should be done, and the results are a wide variety of film styles and ever-changing portrayals of sex.

Some adult filmmakers approach their work as serious artists and writers, some have backgrounds as former (or present) Hollywood cameramen, a few are legit filmmakers who "ended up" in porn, and some know nothing about making films but know what they like to see in sex, and want to make it a reality—these people make up the universe of feature and all-sex filmmakers.

What follows is an alphabetical review list of feature filmmakers: those directors who make films with plot and story line. Just as with sex, the style you like will call to you. For a complete list of each director's films or to find more films made by a director you like (or to avoid ones you don't like), see the index of films by director.

Brad Armstrong

This Wicked studios star director turned a reasonably successful career as a performer into an overnight sensation when he stepped behind the camera and started directing top-notch feature films in 1995. Brad Armstrong still shows up in his films, but who cares what he does when you're totally engrossed in an epic like *Euphoria,* one of the highest-budgeted, most well-written, and damn nearest things to a Hollywood film from the industry to date. He uses big budgets and top stars, though he sometimes pulls starlets out of the low-budget circuits to carry off meaty acting roles—for he has an eye for talent. While the sex scenes are somewhat formulaic and the porn stars look like porn stars, his films are above average for the industry, and he's a talented director worth keeping an eye on.

James Avalon

Cal Vista/Metro's main director James Avalon is a film school graduate who developed some strong notions about what he didn't want to do when making adult films. His main rule is to avoid trite ideas—which shows in the exceptional quality of his outstanding films. A former *Adam Film World* adult movie reviewer, he strives to make films of the caliber that he wanted to see as a reviewer, and is strict about maintaining high production values. Although he is granted high budgets, he will go over budget to ensure that the film is just right. He bucks porn convention by doing things such as editing-in footage to increase emotional intensity or to give the story line depth. His films star high-end actors who don't appear to be porn stars—no mean feat—and his moody, cinematic story-telling envelops the characters so that the performers' acting skills don't appear out of place. And he won't make a film unless he has a strong lead actor—a tactic unheard of in the adult business.

Beautifully shot, timeless, and employing subtlety, Avalon's films open up a whole new direction for the adult feature film—films that are really movies, but with explicit sex. If you're looking for something different, watch an Avalon film.

Chloe

An adult actress with an almost cult-like following of female fans, tiny, brunette, flat-chested Chloe has sex so viscerally, she's got to be seen to be believed. If you've never seen a female orgasm onscreen, just watch one of her films—Chloe says she works in adult film because she likes sex, and that's a tough point to argue once you've watched her eye-popping, thigh-clenching climaxes. A Southern California native, Chloe began work in adult film in 1995, and her take-no-prisoners attitude about pleasure has made fans sit up and take notice. Her penchant for full penetration landed her in the notorious fisting scene in Seymore Butts's (Adam Glasser's) *Tampa Tushy Fest,* which made the news when Glasser was busted for obscenity. Her enthusiasm and enjoyment in the scene probably aided in the "not guilty" ruling. She now directs and stars in her own features, after a short stint of directing and starring in her own all-sex videos. Her all-sex jaunts are fun, raunchy, low-budget wall-to-wall videos, including *Chloe's Catalina Cum-Ons* and *Chloe's "I Came, Did You?"* Chloe is now part of VCA's powerful stable of directors, alongside the legendary Veronica Hart, writing and directing high-budget films that focus on the female sexual experience. Chloe's feature films range from the goofy to the dramatic and star some of the biggest names in the business.

Veronica Hart

Actress-turned-director Veronica Hart created a legacy of unforgettable performances in her brief onscreen career. She now directs multidimensional films that consistently raise the bar for adult feature fare. Hart was one of the first female directors, and like her counterparts she focuses on the female characters and their experience and pleasure, though unlike other female directors she is fearless when she explores the far reaches of female fantasy. Her women like romance, but just as equally demand rough sex, public exhibitionism, and being the gleeful center of attention in down-and-dirty, gang-bang-style scenarios.

Hart spent only a few years performing, but her few films were astoundingly arousing epics—she possessed the raw sexual energy that we always hope we're going to see onscreen, and her acting skills were way above those of her coworkers. Magnetic and alluring, this charming woman quickly left her mark on the industry, winning awards and landing in the XRCO Hall of Fame. She stopped performing in 1984, and picked up the camera to create high-end, plot-driven films that buck the industry's standards and present fantastic, complete films with raw sex in them.

Hart is an in-house director for VCA, and has a casting pool of the best actors in adult, as well as high budgets that she uses to get stunning locations, elaborate sets, great lighting, and stellar cinematography. Her plots are complex, her scripts are tight, and she coaches top-notch actors such as Juli Ashton and Evan Stone to deliver dialogue that naturally comes from their characters. You'll find something near the formula sex scenes in her films, but they're woven into the story line and sometimes show things you wouldn't see in other "couples" feature films, such as female ejaculation. She doesn't waste a moment of her viewer's time, and can show controversial female fantasies such as romantic abduction just as easily as a double-dealing, crime-noir version of the movie *Go,* with overlapping points of view telling the story.

Kris Kramski

A French director whose films reveal extremely high production values, Kris Kramski always elicits amazing performances—especially in the acting—from his performers. He makes films very close in style and feel to Hollywood films, though they contain explicit sex. Sometimes the sex is seamlessly woven into the plot, and sometimes it's glossy, music-video style porn catering to all the expectations of a seasoned porn crowd. While his list is short, a few of the films are quite remarkable, and he has a penchant for working with gorgeous, all-natural female leads who have strong acting chops. His films, which are always shot on 35mm film stock (never video), rarely present much of a plot, but the clean, crisp film style and single-minded focus on the female protagonist's journey introduce an interesting expression of porn that is at once vulnerable and exciting. He takes care to tell a visual story through scene development and camera positioning, edits his footage well so that the film flows, and uses appropriate lighting and atmosphere for each scene. Although his films follow a porn formula for sex, they still are refreshing.

• •

The Busiest Writer You've Never Heard Of: Raven Touchstone

NOT ONLY IS RAVEN TOUCHSTONE a major writer for many of these director's films, she also happens to be a woman. She's an acclaimed photographer (Touchstone is a pseudonym, as if you hadn't guessed) who has been scripting adult films for more than eighteen years. On sets she photographs the actresses, taking stills that are artistic, moody, and dramatic. She doesn't take her scripts particularly seriously—she calls them "light stuff just to get a guy's dick stiff." Her second film was *Just Another Pretty Face* starring Traci Lords, and the third was with the first contract girl, Ginger

Lynn—and she went on to write all fifteen of the Ginger movies for Vivid. In an interview for alicuni.com, she says, "A good porno script is a support system for sex without getting in the way of sex. In other words, the plot holds together and weaves throughout the sex scenes without overpowering them. We don't and can't compete with mainstream films where the whole 120 minutes is plot. Our films and videos run about 90 minutes of which 70 minutes is devoted to sex and the other 20 to story. Consequently, story gets the short end of the stick."

• •

Jonathan Morgan

A performer who won *AVN*'s Best Male Performer of the Year in 1993, Jonathan Morgan began directing in 1997 for Wicked, a porn comedy series, and he also directed a couple of series called *Anal Maniacs* and *Wicked Ways*. His hilarious scripts, with *Young Frankenstein* and *Dr. Strangelove* references, make his films laugh-out-loud funny and great to watch with other people. Some blend a variety of film styles to deliver the full comic effect, and his cast is always populated with strong actors who are top names in the business. Although you're getting porn stars and formula sex, the way he combines them is half the fun. His fun movie-buff approach to film is refreshing, and he uses editing and cinematography well to his advantage to make his videos active and entertaining.

Michael Ninn

The sex-obsessed will draw little solace from the films of Michael Ninn. In them, sex turns lovely lilies into hot-petaled roses of desire, becoming flowers of evil, and the initial manifestations of self-destruction. In my favorite three, the act of copulation drives men and women to madness, good characters become corrupt, the innocent are annihilated, and sex plays second fiddle to its own disastrous implications. His carefully layered tales criticize the porn industry from within and, interestingly, come from a man who has worked for one of the most conventional, big-moneyed companies in the business. And while the mainstream porno behemoth blunders blindly on, fixated on its big dicks and overstuffed tits, Ninn holds up the cynic's mirror and tells us a sex-drenched nightmare of a bedtime story.

Ninn's films bear a strong likeness to the films of Jean Rollin, a late-sixties French director of lesbian vampire films. Most notably, the two directors share the aesthetic of glossy, oddly colored, and eerily-lit Gothic eye-candy, and both portray characters who convey no distinction between right and wrong (and do it poetically). Both have films that are slow-paced, are rife with metaphors communicating story line, and convey a pornographically carnivalesque atmosphere. Their mood is always dark and liquid as the viewer is led through landscapes of sexual compulsion and death. Unlike Rollin's, Ninn's films contain explicit sex, light fetish acts, and your average android porn stars—and exploits their sexual and emotional detachment and blank acting to heighten his creepy, almost gleefully psychotic atmosphere. Bizarre characters, insanity, and unhappy endings are common, and though sometimes the sex steams, it's often so disjointed in context that it drives a wedge between viewer and subject. You walk away with a film-noir taste in your mouth. Nearly all of his films employ a technique that gives the (digital) film a color-saturated, grainy texture, and seems to be missing a few frames per second, giving the whole thing a textured, choppy feel that contributes to the bizarre sexual atmosphere. Ninn's films tend to lack sexual heat, but look absolutely perfect.

In my view, Michael Ninn is one of the most original and unpredictable directors in porn, and has been since his debut in 1992. As his budgets grew, so did the scope of his films, and his films *Sex, Latex,* and *Shock* took porn far beyond the boundaries of adult film, being technically on par with Hollywood film and employing the use of CGI scripts (computer animation) at the same time Hollywood was learning to exploit the technology. Also among his techniques are tricks such as those used in the film *The Matrix,* where he captures sex in "dead time" (also called "bullet time") and the view rotates around slowed-down or frozen action. He works hard to create what he calls "artcore"—artistic hardcore films. It's no wonder, with his style, that he once directed music videos for Capitol Records. He derived his name from the author Anaïs Nin, whose erotic journals were legendary.

Antonio Passolini

With around a dozen directorial credits, Antonio Passolini has managed to make incredible, bizarre, dark, and intense plot-driven films since his debut in 1998. Lots of money and thought go into a "Passolini Transmission," and when you watch one you can expect high production values, high-gloss visuals, a variety of film styles, and top names in the porn biz making the most of the loosely followed formula sex scenes. His films focus on human vulnerability and can be complex human dramas, surreal jaunts into hell, or fiercely critical parodies of the adult industry. His films are smart and well-acted, he tends to use the usual cadre of big-name actors and enhanced starlets, and his timing can sometimes (not always) become plodding and drag out through long monologues.

Passolini's first incarnation in the adult industry was as a writer. He developed and wrote the Caballero hit *Stiff Competition* under the name Colin DeTacqu, later adopting the name Johnny Jump-Up to write numerous Dark Bros. classics including *Black Throat* and *Devil in Miss Jones 3 & 4.* Before embarking on his own directorial career, Passolini was the executive producer and writer of Michael Ninn's seminal works, *Latex* and *Shock,* and ran interference with VCA directors as a producer.

Passolini made his debut as a director with *Café Flesh 2,* which garnered wide critical praise and won the 1998 *AVN* "Best Video Feature" award. His second video opus, *Devil in Miss Jones 6,* was a top-renting tape in 1999. His dark, dramatic feature *Bliss* departs from his quirky style and delivers many blistering, emotionally driven sex scenes.

Michael Raven

Active as a director since 1998, Michael Raven had a small stint as a performer from 1999 to 2001 and continues to direct high-quality story- and character-driven videos. Sin City's resident ace director, he has decent budgets to throw around on a variety of projects, from soft-focus, romantic couples'–market fare to mafia crime films and even retellings of Milton's *Paradise Lost.* His films range from slightly overdone (perhaps intentionally?) to well-shot porn with a story to tie the action together, though he has done some all-sex films as well.

Candida Royalle

Another performer-turned-director, Candida Royalle made her mark by creating some of the very first porn made specifically with female viewers in mind. Coming from a pro-porn feminist perspective, Royalle felt that women rejected adult videos because their fantasies and needs weren't being addressed, so she created Femme Productions in 1984 with the goal of offering erotic films from Royalle's idea of a woman's perspective and presenting positive sexual-role modeling. The result has been more than a dozen films that concentrate on story and character, even a few runaway best-sellers. The first spate of her films verged on soft core, though gradually they have become more explicit and include a wider breadth of sex acts, such as anal sex.

While attending art school, pretty Royalle worked as a figure model to earn some extra cash, and became one of the top nude models in the nation, posing for scores of men's magazines. At the time, the burgeoning world of 1970s porn—plus the lure of more money—was calling to many erotic dancers and models, and Royalle was one of the many who answered. Since then, she's been a major figure in the adult film industry, and in 1975 got off to an explosive start as the lead character in *The Analyst,* a very early exploration of the appeal of anal sex. Her steamy sensuality won over fans and critics alike, and she was soon one of the most sought-after female performers. She turned in more than fifty scorching performances, including turns in the XRCO Hall of Fame films *Femmes De Sade, Outlaw Ladies,* and *Sexcapades.*

In the early 1980s, Royalle took her talents behind the camera and wrote the legendary porn flick *Blue Magic.* Her films are well-shot and have great acting with big-name, well-liked porn stars such as Missy, Mickey G, Nina Hartley, and Mark Davis. The stories are cute and romantic, though there are often long gaps in timing that can leave the viewer feeling stranded while the camera rolls. The sex in Royalle's films is always packed with chemistry, and though her films contain the explicit sex that porn viewers expect, it is presented in a more realistic light (that is, with internal ejaculation and a lack of gynecological close-ups). A few of her films show anal sex. Because they present a female perspective, intertwine plot and sex, and feature sex not of the brightly lit, hard-core variety, her films are routinely recommended for couples new to adult film.

Paul Thomas

With more than 200 feature productions under his belt, countless awards for his films, multiple XRCO Hall of Fame awards, and a reputation as a paradigmatic feature director in porn, Paul Thomas is the Scorsese of adult film. Thomas takes his big budgets and sculpts them into fully realized, plot-driven vehicles. In his films the best actors in the business push character development to the limit, the sex is woven into the script, the plot and dialogue are unpredictable and well-crafted, and the cinematography is above and beyond porn fare. Paul Thomas makes *movies*.

Directing is Thomas's natural skill, but it wasn't his first experience in the industry. He began as a performer, a favorite star from the golden age of porn. He was born in 1951 in Winnetka, Illinois, the son of wealthy parents and the nephew of baked-goods queen Sara Lee. He studied political science at the University of Wisconsin at Madison, then felt his calling was acting and moved to New York City. Attractive and talented, he soon starred in the Broadway production of *Hair*, landed the role of Peter in the film version of *Jesus Christ Superstar*, then moved to Los Angeles to pursue his acting career. He met with much success, getting roles in TV series such as *Police Story* and *Mannix*, but soon tired of the L.A. meat grinder. In 1974 he found himself in San Francisco, in a production of the musical spoof *Beach Blanket Bingo*, when he met porn impresarios the Mitchell Brothers. They convinced him to perform for them, and in 1976 he made his debut in *The Autobiography of a Flea*.

After a wild ride through the 1970s porn scene, several relationships with famous actresses such as Annete Haven and Veronica Hart, and a stint in jail for smuggling cocaine, Thomas found his natural role behind the camera. His first production was *Robofox* in 1988, coproduced with Henri Pachard. Since then, his style has evolved beyond the standards of contemporary porn features, with his focus on noir themes, twist-and-turn plots, and stories that revolve around the frailties of the human condition.

His movies are seldom "feel-good" films, for they often contain murder, betrayal, and unhappy endings. They are mature, however, in that they do not present a pastiche of "safe" and predictable story arcs. In them, men fall in love with self-destructive sex workers, wanna-be porn directors are fooled into committing murder for the entertainment of those with more experience, and, always, everyone is out for himself. Paul Thomas is the in-house director for Vivid, spending its big budgets well, sometimes using real film stock, and shooting elaborate period pieces on location.

Tina Tyler

Canadian-born Tina Tyler, one of the hottest femmes in the business, is another supremely skilled performer-turned-director, and she's only just begun. Her feature film *Tina Tyler's Going Down* is a runaway best-seller, with excellent production values, terrific editing, and sex woven expertly into a clever plot. Tyler was born in 1965, and since her 1992 debut in adult she's had a loyal following of female fans and male fans of bisexual films. She has also directed and compiled all-sex videos that are her choicest cuts of girl–girl scenes and lip-licking blow-job scenes. The future looks bright for the films of this smart, beautiful woman.

Michael Zen

Since 1977 Michael Zen has been hard at work directing feature porn, and though adult films are made quickly he has not hurried himself and has only made some eighty films in his time. While he has done a couple of all-sex series, the majority of his films are plot driven, with production values ranging from medium, with poor premises, typical talent, and rough sets, to high, with amazing performances and great atmosphere (such as *Bawdy and Soul*). A Zen film gives you a good evening of porn, with enough plot to tie the formulaic scenes together.

Feature Film Reviews

The videos listed in this chapter are feature films hand-picked for their exceptional popularity with viewers and high marks in all categories—as well as being favorites of reviewers and having a focus on female pleasure. These are the films with higher production values, better story lines and concepts, and top-rate acting. Some verge on soft core, while most of the others contain the customary formula and close-up camerawork that denotes usual porn production values. Many of these deviate, however, from the norm—these are the best feature films.

Porn surpasses itself when it tells contemporary stories, set in the here-and-now, using themes intimate to the industry. The viewer should always take into account porn's narcissism, and never forget the bottom line—that these films are intended for masturbation or to ignite arousal with a lover. And these delicious, arousing films do just that. I think you'll be pleasantly surprised at the quality and diversity today's directors have to offer.

Affairs of the Heart

The minimal plot centers on a woman's flashbacks to her hottest and most romantic sexual encounters in her relationship. The terrific sex scenes show passionate sex that includes concrete focus between the performers, and cuddling.

DIRECTOR: Bud Lee, 1993, 79 min.

CAST: Alex Jordan, Brittany O'Connell, Lene Hefner, Tina Tyler, Jon Dough, Marc Davis, Nick East

America XXX: A Tribute to Sex & Rock and Roll

In this slick Hustler video, a rotating series of question-and-answer sessions surround rock music videos that are composed of politically thematic explicit sex. Chloe asks the questions, and Larry Flynt and a number of unknown L.A. rock bands answer with opinions on subjects ranging from porn and obscenity to the death penalty and AIDS. Glossy, well-shot music videos put to each band's music contain formulaic and uninspired sex, though the Flint answers are as always, interesting and compelling. The ignorance of the L.A. rockers and porn auteur Johnny Toxic on issues such as AIDS is eye-opening.

DIRECTOR: Kris Kramski, 2002, 71 min.

CAST: Chloe (nonsex), Christal, Claudia, Erika, Giu Sky, Monica Moore, Oana, Sheila Scott, Sophia Marquez, Zsophia, Alex, Chris Mountain, Johnny Toxic, Larry Flynt, Lucky, Renato

NOTE: Chloe is in a nonsex role.

Woman Penetrates Man

Natural Cast

Unsightly Boob Job

Well-Made Film

Real Female Orgasm

An American Girl in Paris

Low on plot but high in production values and explosive and outrageous sex scenes, the video centers on a lonely American girl in Paris, who, like, wow, who could've guessed, loses her wallet, must survive *somehow,* and basically has really fantastic sex on her vacation, making those of us who just saw the Louvre feel a little let down. This is a stellar sex film, and though the scene setups don't always make sense in reality, it's all shot entirely on location in beautiful Paris, with great lighting and an attractive cast.

DIRECTOR: Kris Kramski, 1998, 69 min.

CAST: Brooke, Coralie, Karen Lancaume, Lucie Morgan, Patrice Cabanel, Bruno Assix, Dino Toscani, Fred Thomas

Anal Nurses

Oh, you've just got to love the title of this film: so subtle. But the goofy title belies a great video, set in a hospital where a couple's relationship goes awry as they second-guess each other's infidelities, creating the premise for loads of hot anal sex in a hospital setting. Insert all your "turn your head and cough" jokes here. This tape is fun for so many reasons: skimpy nurse uniforms, beautiful female Asian performers in the cast, a reality-TV style narrative format, heated anal sex couples-style.

DIRECTOR: Penny Nichols, 2002, 85 min.

CAST: Dru Berrymore, Fujiko Kano, Jewels Jade, Maliccia, Phyllisha Anne, Chris Cannon, Ted Hunter, Joel Lawrence, Rafe, Tony Tedeschi

Anything That Moves

One of Leslie's early directorial efforts, with a focus on two strippers gone on a sexual rampage, à la *Thelma and Louise.* Plenty of erotic dancing, good dialogue and delivery, and passionate sex. Read about John Leslie in Chapter 8, "All Sex, No Plot."

DIRECTOR: John Leslie, 1992, 76 min.

CAST: Cassidy, Denise Lynn Roberts (nonsex), Flame (nonsex), Heidi Kat, Kristine Shap (nonsex), Melody Moore (nonsex), Sharon Driver (nonsex), Shanna Rose (nonsex), Selena Steele, Teri Diver (nonsex), Tianna Taylor (nonsex), Traci Winn, Joel Clupper, Steve Hatcher (nonsex), Lee Chandler (nonsex), Nick East, Nick Santiago, Randy Spears, Steve Drake, Tim Lake, Tony Tedeschi (nonsex)

| Dominant Women | Violet's Top Choice | Intense Chemistry | Extreme Sex Acts | Great for Newbies |

Appassionata

In a role that is porn imitating life as life imitates porn, Asia Carrera plays a young classical pianist reincarnated. Carrera showcases her talents as not only a trained pianist but also a passionate actress in this much-loved, highly praised film.

DIRECTOR: Asia Carrera; Bud Lee, 1998, 92 min.

CAST: Asia Carrera, Avalon, Brittany Andrews, Charlie, Holly Body, Johnni Black, Leanna Heart, Laura Palmer, Lisa Harper, Raylene, Roxanne Hall, Sindee Coxx, Veronica Hart (nonsex), Alec Metro, Alex Sanders, John Decker, Jonathan Morgan, Steve Hatcher, Marc Davis

Ashlyn Rising

See why Ashlyn Gere is such a notable sex performer in this story of a woman who regains her self-esteem through sexual adventures. After a steamy opener with her crass boyfriend Rocco Siffredi and his "beer buddy," Siffredi leaves her and she's devastated, until she sees her prosex therapist who has some very titil-lating prescriptions, including that Gere act as a voyeur to live sex. Includes a sweet seduction of Gere by everyone's dream therapist Nina Hartley, a sizzling peep-show-booth encounter, and features great sex scenes all-around, told from the female character's perspective.

DIRECTOR: Layne Parker, 1995, 88 min.

CAST: Ashlyn Gere, Anna Malle, Nina Hartley, Tera Heart, Colt Steel, Hank Armstrong, Marc Davis, Rocco Siffredi, Sean Michaels

Babylon

Blonde starlet Lexus is the downtrodden niece of evil oversexed aunt Jeanna Fine, and fantasy trumps reality as both slip into a fantasy world as in *Alice in Wonderland*. Our Alice has lots of sex in bizarre and strange situations while try-ing to escape Fine, but Alice gets the last laugh when auntie's selfishness lands her in a sort of sexual purgatory.

DIRECTOR: Michael Zen, 1999, 120 min.

CAST: Candy Apples, Chloe, Dee, Halli Aston, Inari Vachs, Janine, Jeanna Fine, Jill Kelly, Kobe Tai, Lexus Locklear, Bobby Vitale, Johnny Appleseed, Jake Steed, Michael J. Cox, Tony Tedeschi, Vince Voyeur

NOTE: Contains a sex machine.

Woman Penetrates Man	Natural Cast	Unsightly Boob Job	Well-Made Film	Real Female Orgasm

Back and Beyond

This is a great summer-release-style haunted house flick, but populated with professional sex performers. Years ago, a group of friends went to an abandoned estate to party, and one of them drowned in the pond while everyone else was oblivious. Turns out those meddling kids are still partying at the estate, and a present-day group arrives for some creepy fun and is treated to haunting and sexing from beyond.

DIRECTOR: Nic Cramer, 1998, 74 min.

CAST: Alyssa Allure, Blair Segal, Chloe, Caroline Pierce, Goldie McHawn, John Decker, Brick Majors, Brian Surewood, Ian Daniels, John West

Bad Wives

Two wives are bored with the ball-and-chain of married life and discover the delights of infidelity and raunchy sex at the hands of a grocery checkout boy played by Steven St. Croix. The performance by Melissa Hill is excellent, and scenes include—you guessed it—supermarket counters and a very staged scene à la *The Cook, The Thief, His Wife and Her Lover* in a meat locker, though not as macabre.

DIRECTOR: Paul Thomas, 1997, 147 min.

CAST: Dyanna Lauren, Melissa Hill, Missy, Stephanie Swift, Tricia Devereaux, Jon Dough, Mickey G (nonsex), Steven St. Croix, Tony Tedeschi

NOTE: High ratings from *AVN Magazine*, won an *AVN* award in 1997, lots of anal sex.

Bad Wives 2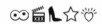

Different wives, but they're in a lot of trouble this time. In prison for trying to murder their deceitful husbands, two wives are tempted and released by the devil, played to the hilt by Randy Spears. Turns out the gals are innocent, but the devil does everything he can to tempt them into offing the jerks for real, in an effort to get them onto the dark side. Great film, with a terrific masturbation scene and a torrid sex scene between then-married couple Ava Vincent and John Decker.

DIRECTOR: Paul Thomas, 2001, 106 min.

CAST: Angel Desirees, April Flowers, Casey, Jolene, Ava Vincent, Kylie Ireland, Mariesa, Raylene, Rea'l Good, Ryan Conner, Sirena Scott, Shelbee Myne, Alec Metro, John Decker, Bobby Vitale, Erik Everhard, Eric Price, Hershel Savage, Jason McCain, Randy Spears

NOTE: Contains a gory murder scene, won an *AVN* award.

| Dominant Women | Violet's Top Choice | Intense Chemistry | Extreme Sex Acts | Great for Newbies |

Bawdy and Soul

Yup, it's a porn spoof on the movie *Ghost*. To help a woman find the murderer of her private detective boyfriend, Asia Carrera channels the boyfriend and they uncover the mystery, but not before everyone gets to have a lot of sex. The crime and sex with ghosts theme is a tried-and-true staple in porn, but this video is above the rest with terrific casting and several marvelous sex scenes—especially with Chloe's otherworldly orgasms.

DIRECTOR: Michael Zen, 1998, 81 min.

CAST: Asia Carrera, Chloe, Holli Woods, Johnni Black, Lene Hefner, Shelbee Myne, Jonathan Morgan, Marc Davis

Believe It Or Not; Believe It Or Not 2

High production values are purposely tweaked to look lowbrow as director Thomas takes adult actresses, hooks them to a lie detector, and gets them to confess their hottest/craziest sexual encounters—then has them reenact the scenarios for the camera. Some are true and some are made up—can you tell which ones? A fun premise for great sex.

Believe It Or Not

DIRECTOR: Paul Thomas, 2001, 106 min.

CAST: Cassidey, Brooke Hunter, Dayton Rain, Ava Vincent, Mariesa, Nikita Denise, Zana, Alec Metro (nonsex), John Decker, Dale DaBone, Don Hollywood (nonsex), Jason McCain, Joey Ray, Mark Wood, Steve Taylor, T. J. Cummings

NOTE: Ava Vincent has a scene with her then-fiancé, John Decker.

Believe It Or Not 2

DIRECTOR: Paul Thomas, 2001, 70 min.

CAST: Cassidey, Dayton Rain, Heather Lyn, Tabitha Stern, Alec Metro, Dillion Day, Eric Masterson, Jason McCain, Joey Ray, Jonathan Stern, Manny Trio, Tony Tedeschi, Vince Voyeur

Woman Penetrates Man

Natural Cast

Unsightly Boob Job

Well-Made Film

Real Female Orgasm

Betty Bleu

The only thing this energetic sexfest has in common with the foreign film *Betty Blue* is that it's from France; other than that it's a forties-era period piece cast with attractive European actors in great costumes and sets. On par with a European feature film release, it had an unheard-of budget ($250,000) and was shot entirely on location in Florence, Italy, and Paris, France. Great plot, marred by bad dubbing.

DIRECTOR: Alex Perry, 1996, 80 min.

CAST: Anita Rinaldi, Tania Laiviere, Eros Christaldi, Jennifer Diore, Lea Martini, Michelle, Maria DeSanchez, Herve Pierre Gustave, Fancesco Malcom, Oliver Sanchez

NOTE: Foreign release. No safer sex.

Bliss

The tension is palpable in Passolini's filmic comment on what normal people are really like. Outstanding acting and innovative camerawork make it feel almost too real, but the kicker is the compelling story line in which porn star Juli Ashton's straight, perfect-wife character becomes the center of all the unraveling relationships in her life as a result of her sexual compulsiveness. You'll find no dull moments here, from characters you really feel for (or despise) getting blow jobs on the sly to a show-stopping, kinky anal sex encounter with Chloe, known for her trademark authentic explosive onscreen orgasms. Yes, the actors all appear to be baby-boomers—that seems to be the point—but here we can see the shadows that they can't deal with, we become wet by the desperate and furtive quality of their sexual encounters, while the whole film seems even to be shot in the shadows.

DIRECTOR: Antonio Passolini, 1999, 120 min.

CAST: Chloe, Gina Ryder, Juli Ashton, Nikita, Tina Tyler, Joel Lawrence, Steve Hatcher, Tony Tedeschi

Dominant Women	Violet's Top Choice	Intense Chemistry	Extreme Sex Acts	Great for Newbies

Blue Movie

In a well-executed and highly praised comedy, Jenna Jameson is a spunky female reporter out to get a story in the bizarre world of the adult film industry, and winds up starring in sex films weirder than even the ones made in reality. Features a hilarious Steven St. Croix in Carmen Miranda drag throughout the film, great visuals, and oodles of very hot sex, especially the early cunnilingus scene with St. Croix. A big-budget feature that's more sophisticated than other porn attempts at comedy.

DIRECTOR: Michael Zen, 1995, 83 min.

CAST: Dallas, Jackie Beat (nonsex), Jeanna Fine, Jenna Jameson, Jordan St. James, Lana Sands, Rebecca Lord, Tera Heart, Alex Sanders, Steven St. Croix, TT Boy, Tony Tedeschi

NOTE: Won several *AVN* awards in 1995.

Bobby Sox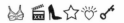

One of Thomas's most perfect films and one of the most complete films containing sex ever made. Follow monster-movie actor Jeremy Dayton into a small town to promote his latest B-movie effort—where a little sexual shakeup with Nikki Tyler unearths a whole lot of repressed sexual energy. Great acting and an excellent, witty script give depth to terrific characters, including a troublemaking teenager and a dissatisfied dominatrix, in addition to delicious nonformula sex scenes such as a juicy movie-theater encounter with a masturbating voyeur.

DIRECTOR: Paul Thomas, 1996, 144 min.

CAST: Chelsea Blue, Chloe, Jenteal, Kimberly Kummings, Madelyn Night (nonsex), Shanna McCullough, Nikki Tyler, Alex Sanders, Bobby Vitale, Jay Ashley, Jon Dough, Jamie Gillis, Steven St. Croix, TT Boy

NOTE: Contains a male submission scene, no safer sex, received a "perfect 10" from *AVN Magazine*.

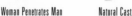

| Woman Penetrates Man | Natural Cast | Unsightly Boob Job | Well-Made Film | Real Female Orgasm |

Borderline

Infidelity is the central theme in this film, which explores the disastrous exploits of two cheating lovers who go to Mexico to "make it official" and be together. They become stranded in a small town when their car breaks down and they realize they've made a mistake—but the unusual result is lots of tense, fiery sex. A great, wonderfully made dramatic film (with unpredictable twists) shot on location in Mexico amidst beautiful scenery.

DIRECTOR: Paul Thomas, 1995, 118 min.

CAST: Alexis DeVell (nonsex), Alabama, Alicia Rio, Bridgette Monroe, Celeste, Coco Lee (nonsex), Dorian Grant, Felecia, Jill Kelly, Madelyn Night, Missy, Nici Sterling, Tabitha, Tyffany Million, Bobby Vitale, Guy DaSilva, Gino Grant, George Kaplan (nonsex), Hector Gomez (nonsex), Marc Davis, Steven St. Croix, Tony Montana

NOTE: Won an *AVN* award in 1995.

The Bridal Shower

Five women confess their sexual exploits at a bridal shower, and we get to see the exploits in several high-caliber, well-acted vignettes. All focusing on female experience, the scenes include food play, blindfolds, and a demure Nina Hartley learning to strip to seduce her lover.

DIRECTOR: Candida Royalle, 1997, 80 min.

CAST: Sharon Kane, Nina Hartley, Melissa Hill, Missy, Porsche Lynn, Guy DaSilva, Jonathan Morgan, John Curtis, Mike Horner, Mickey G

NOTE: First three-way in a Royalle film, no anal.

Dominant Women　　Violet's Top Choice　　Intense Chemistry　　Extreme Sex Acts　　Great for Newbies

Bride of Double Feature

Following the same format as *Double Feature*, this film treats us to two more pur- posely B-grade spoofs from "Cheesy Pictures," the first a dry-witted porn treatment of *A Shot in the Dark* and the second a jungle-movie lampoon featur- ing Randy Spears as "Momo the Jungle Boy." High weirdness mixes with the plot's pacing problems to make a surreal porn flick, though the all-star cast, excellent sex performances, and acting talents of Spears, Serenity, and Asia Carrera make it a fun, lighthearted sex flick.

DIRECTOR: Jonathan Morgan, 2000, 115 min.

CAST: Serenity, Tabitha Stevens, Bridgette Kerkove, Asia Carrera, Tasha Hunter, Anji Cooper, Daniella Rush, Kaylin, Randy Spears, Mickey G, Mike Horner, Kyle Stone, Dave Hardman, Anthony Crane

Buda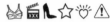

For Rocco Siffredi and John (Buttman) Stagliano fans, this three-hour-plus crime drama is a must-have. Buda is the capital city in Eastern Europe that became one with another city, Pest, to become Budapest, which is essentially Porn Valley's sis- ter city—the place in Europe where most porn is cast and shot. Buttman takes advantage of the ample-assed talent pool and pits Rocco as the man caught in the middle of an Eastern European gang war, centering on a runaway gangster's girl- friend—who gets saved by Rocco. Lots of smart plot twists and extra-long, extremely hard-driving sex scenes, and lots of poetic, lingering shots of beautiful butts. Read about John "Buttman" Stagliano in Chapter 8, "All Sex, No Plot."

DIRECTOR: John Stagliano, 1997, 90 min.

CAST: Chrissy Ann, Zenza Raggi, Angela, Suzy, Ursula Moore, Sylvia, Holly Black, Amanda Steel, Sophia, Christy, Blondy, Reka, Judith Grant, Emanuel, Zsolt Walton, Andrew Youngman, Mike Foster, Steve Hard, Cowboy, Cho-Cho, Joe Koo, Marlon Xtravaganza, Leslie, Randy Spears, John Stagliano, Rocco Siffredi

NOTE: Foreign release. Won an *AVN* award in 1998.

| Woman Penetrates Man | Natural Cast | Unsightly Boob Job | Well-Made Film | Real Female Orgasm |

Cabin Fever

A woman goes on a retreat to a cabin in the woods to find privacy and have time to focus on her artwork, but the surprise addition of a handsome handyman changes everything—especially when their unusual courtship begins. Good production values, with a focus on the female point of view and female pleasure.

DIRECTOR: Deborah Shames, 1995, 45 min.

CAST: Judd Dunning and Belinda Farrell

NOTE: Independent filmmaker. Soft core with an edge; no genital close-ups, anal, or facial ejaculation.

Cabin Fever

Not to be confused with the feminist soft-core porn film above, this great film nevertheless earns high marks. Three gal-pals run out of gas in the mountains, and hike to a nearby cabin to spend the night. One clever scene follows another as the cabin's male owner comes home, an errant handyman is seduced, a snowboarder crashes in, everyone's mad girlfriends show up, and sex on the sly becomes the order of the day. A complex, clever story that the sex fits quite naturally.

DIRECTOR: Jim Powers, 1995, 82 min.

CAST: Baily, Fallon, Heather Lee, Olivia, Shelly Lyons, Dick Nasty, Gerry Pike, Kyle Stone

Café Flesh 2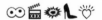

Outstanding visuals, bizarre atmosphere and themes, and mesmerizing sex scenes make this sequel to the classic *Café Flesh* (see Chapter 7) a film in its own right. Jeanna Fine is the proprietor of the legendary café of the future, whose stage shows deliver explicit sex to a sexually incapable audience. Terrific, though bizarre and often wacky, sex.

DIRECTOR: Antonio Passolini, 1998, 135 min.

CAST: Jeanna Fine, Kitten Natividad (nonsex), Raylene, Rebecca Lord, Sally Layd, Stacy Valentine, Veronica Hart (nonsex), Alec Metro, John Decker, Billy Glyde, Brian Surewood, David Hardman, Simon Delo (nonsex), TT Boy, Tony Tedeschi, Vince Voyeur

NOTE: Contains a scene with mimes, and won *AVN*'s Best Video award in 1998.

| Dominant Women | Violet's Top Choice | Intense Chemistry | Extreme Sex Acts | Great for Newbies |

Chameleons (Not the Sequel)

This early John Leslie feature explores the possibilities of being able to change into any body imaginable and then have sex. Energetic sex, with great performances throughout.

DIRECTOR: John Leslie, 1992, 95 min.

CAST: Ashlyn Gere, Brandy Alexandre (nonsex), Carolyn Monroe (nonsex), Deidre Holland, Fawn Miller, Leanna Foxxx, P. J. Sparxx, Sunset Thomas, Traci Winn, Don Fernando (nonsex), Jon Dough, Micky Ray, Nick East, Nick Rage (nonsex), Rocco Siffredi, Tim Lake, Woody Long, Zack Thomas

NOTE: Won an *AVN* award in 1992.

Chloe: A Day at the Beach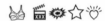

High production values and great cinematography are the frame for a very dark tale of a woman (Chloe) who is addicted to sexual submission and degradation. The gritty, character-driven plot contains emotionally difficult sex scenes that many viewers might find disturbing—especially because they fuel the myth of sex addiction. Chloe has many incredible orgasms; it's a very unconventional, plot-heavy adult film, though definitely not a "feel good" film.

DIRECTOR: Kris Kramski, 1999, 120 min.

CAST: Barett Moore, Chloe, Danielle Rodgers, Cheyenne Silver, Chris Cannon, James Bonn, Randy Spears

NOTE: No safer sex; Chloe, however, did have the entire cast get full-panel STD and HIV tests to ensure safety (while maintaining the realism of the characters' condomless sex).

Christine's Secret

A woman wants to escape big-city life and is looking for love, so she goes to a country inn, where she finds both. Realistic, passionate sex, non–porn star bodies, and a lovely location are the high notes, though the bad music is distracting.

DIRECTOR: Candida Royalle, 1986, 75 min.

CAST: Carol Cross, Chelsea Blake, Taija Rae, Marita Ekberg, Joey Silvera, Jake West, George Payne, Anthony Casino

NOTE: Internal ejaculations and no facials, one external come shot, no anal.

Woman Penetrates Man	Natural Cast	Unsightly Boob Job	Well-Made Film	Real Female Orgasm

Clockwork Orgy

Kubrick might have enjoyed this serious tribute to his legendary film *Clockwork Orange,* for it turns the tables on gender and sets a gang of cruel, horny women roaming the streets taking sex from whom they please—often without consent. It's all about female power and satisfaction, and the performers run with the sexual energy, taking it to the limit.

DIRECTOR: Nic Cramer, 1996, 75 min.

CAST: Isis Nile, Kaitlyn Ashley, Kitty Yung (nonsex), Nicole Lace, Olivia, Rebecca Lord, Shelby Stevens, Alex Sanders, Dick Nasty, Jay Ashley (nonsex), Jon Dough, Jonathan Morgan, Kyle Stone, Steve Austin (nonsex), Vince Voyeur

Club Hades

Kinky S/M nightspot Club Hades is the setting for female tattoo artist Missy's seduction at the hands of her best friend's boyfriend. Great sex and attention to S/M and fetish detail make this a notable film. Read more about Ernest Greene in Chapter 9, "S/M Features."

DIRECTOR: Ernest Greene, 1997, 71 min.

CAST: Ariana, Chloe, Leanna Heart, Missy, Roxanne Hall, Alex Sanders, John Decker, Marc Davis, Marc Wallice

NOTE: S/M activities with sex.

Club Sin

Deciding that their divorcée support group is too wimpy, two women start an underground sex club similar to the film *Fight Club* where men are used as a sexual proving ground for the predatory women. Well shot and acted, with a refreshing take on women taking satisfaction from—and being tougher than—the men for each other's sake, rather than to "get a man."

DIRECTOR: Antonio Passolini, 2001, 99 min.

CAST: Ashlyn Gere, Brooke Hunter, Chloe, Gwen Summers, Kiki D'Aire, Kylie Ireland, Shay Sights, Chris Cannon, Cheyne Collins, Dillion Day, Evan Stone, Ian Daniels, Steve Hatcher, Kyle Stone, Lee Stone, Nick Manning, Pat Myne

Dominant Women	Violet's Top Choice	Intense Chemistry	Extreme Sex Acts	Great for Newbies

Conquest

Vengeance, action, sex, love and the ways of pirates on the high seas are what this fantastic film is all about—and this film shines in every category. While it's easy to imagine all the ways a porn film could butcher the pirate premise, this complete film does it justice, with real ships, island locations, complex character motivations, and stars who can pull it all off. The cinematography is excellent, fight scenes are choreographed nicely, and the fiery, passionate sex belongs in the story line. In this epic, a pirate captain seeks revenge on the man who killed his love, and as he sets out, he discovers a captivating stowaway who seeks revenge on the same villain, while a mad prince seeks to eliminate them both. The sex is intense but not nasty, in fact there isn't even the hint of kink, and those new to porn will feel comfortable with the sexual contextualizing.

DIRECTOR: Brad Armstrong, 1996, 115 min.

CAST: Alex Dane, Asia Carrera, Jenna Jameson, Juli Ashton, Julie Rage (nonsex), Kia, Missy, Sahara Sands, Shayla LaVeaux, Alex Sanders, Bobby Vitale, Brad Armstrong, Claudio, Dic Tracy (nonsex), E Z Ryder (nonsex), Marc Davis, Mickey G, Sean Rider, Tom Byron, Vince Voyeur

NOTE: Shot on film.

Corporate Assets 2

Juli Ashton is the wife trying to leave behind her wild past as a sex worker and live in the country, but when a group of their old friends show up, her husband's libido goes out of bounds and hers goes off the scale. Gorgeous pairing of Mark Davis and Ashton, who can really act, and the sex gets pretty kinky as they explore their "darker" fantasies, including candle wax, female submission, and a great group scene.

DIRECTOR: Thomas Paine, 1997, 95 min.

CAST: Asia Carrera, Chloe, Nina Hartley, Heaven Lee, Juli Ashton, Jeanna Fine, Johnni Black, Rebecca Lord, Shayla LaVeaux, Alex Sanders, John Decker, Steve Hatcher, Mark Davis, Michael J. Cox

| Woman Penetrates Man | Natural Cast | Unsightly Boob Job | Well-Made Film | Real Female Orgasm |

The Creasemaster's Wife

Tyffany Million is the beleaguered former wife of the man known as "The Creasemaster," obsessed with her—and other women's—labial folds. She's free thanks to the divorce, but the whole experience has made her a little nuts, and when a pair of friends take her in and try to introduce her to some nice men, she scares them off one by one with her wackadoo sexual aggression. The film is told through a flashback interview format with the couple, and the overall quality is high.

DIRECTOR: Gregory Dark (the Dark Bros.), 1993, 80 min.

CAST: Tiffany Mynx, Sierra, Tyffany Million, Leanna Foxxx, Jaclynn Kitty, Devon Shire, Tyffany Million, Danielle Rogers, Steve Drake, Jonathan Morgan, Tom Byron, Randy Spears, Mike Horner

Curse of the Catwoman

This is a reviewer and fan favorite, largely for the hot hot sex, scorching masturbation scene, and eerie, moody lighting and cinematography. In a great drama about a female-dominant tribe, two women portray the habits of cats in heat and their predatory ways. Sounds strange, but hey, it's the early nineties, they have big hair, and it's really pretty cool.

DIRECTOR: John Leslie, 1991, 85 min.

CAST: Kathleen Jentry, Zara Whites, Patricia Kennedy, Raven, Racquel Darrian, Ashly Nicole, Derek Lane, TT Boy, Jamie Gillis, Randy Spears, John Stagliano, Marc Wallice

NOTE: Won an *AVN* award in 1991.

Dangerous Games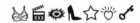

Talk about explosive sex—the first scene throws you head first into the most gritty, intense coupling you'd imagine, and with the dark plot to fuel the tension, the film and seamlessly woven sex scenes only get better from there. Chloe is a woman who is desperate for a way out, and plots a double-deal with characters even shadier than she suspects. A thrilling neo-noir film, standing head and shoulders above the rest.

DIRECTOR: Veronica Hart, 2001, 118 min.

CAST: Chloe, Jade Marcela, Keri Windsor, Mia Smiles, Tina Tyler, Billy Glyde, Ian Daniels, Steve Hatcher, Kyle Stone, Mickey G

Dominant Women	Violet's Top Choice	Intense Chemistry	Extreme Sex Acts	Great for Newbies

Dark Angels

In this B-grade, though entertaining, female vampire film, innocent Jewel D'Nyle stumbles across a bloody murder and winds up the target of evil vampire queen Sydnee Steele. She thinks her flatfoot boyfriend can protect her, but she's wrong, and dream sequences overlap with her reality as she discovers she's become one of them. Hokey L.A. outfits, but decent porn formula sex.

DIRECTOR: Nic Andrews, 2000, 118 min.

CAST: April Flowers, Delaney Daniels (nonsex), Felecia Ryder, Ginger Paige, Jewel De'Nyle, Justine Romee (nonsex), McKayla, Miko Lee (nonsex), Nancy V (nonsex), Paige Sinclair (nonsex), Sydnee Steele, Andre Madness (nonsex), Dillion Day, Erik Everhard, Evan Stone (nonsex), George Kaplan (nonsex), Mike Horner, Mickey G, VooDoo Child

NOTE: Winner of six *AVN* awards.

Dark Garden

Dark and dreamlike, with very textured visuals, this film has a misguided cop investigating a pair of magnetic but insane twin brothers who are plotting to rule the world with a device that creates and fuels sex addiction. Twisted and neo-noir, but each scene is slick as a music video.

DIRECTOR: Michael Ninn, 1999, 115 min.

CAST: Vicca, Lea Martini, Mia Smiles, Nikita, Juli Ashton, Julian, Lisa Belle, Michael J. Coxx, Ramon, John Decker, Tyce Bune, Jack Garfield

NOTE: Won several *AVN* awards in 1999.

Debbie Does Dallas '99

In a modern departure from the classic, a group of basketball cheerleaders needs cash to buy a bus and decides the best way to get money fast is to try their hands—and everything else—at stripping. Cute, fun, and smart, this film show-cases a bunch of gals having fun taking it off and taking on rival teams, making a perfect opportunity for group scenes.

DIRECTOR: Paul Thomas, 1999, 82 min.

CAST: Stephanie Swift, Lovette, Mickey Lynn, Raina, Vince Voyeur, Mr. Marcus, Tony Tedeschi, Mark Davis

    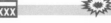

Woman Penetrates Man   Natural Cast   Unsightly Boob Job   Well-Made Film   Real Female Orgasm

Decadence

Ashlyn Gere and Victoria Paris star as lovers who take a walk down memory lane and retell their sexual adventures. The elaborate fantasies include two women taking their pleasure from a restrained man under a waterfall and a totally outrageous and, yes, decadent group scene. Ninn's trademark disjointed (though mesmerizing) visual storytelling and camerawork add to the visual eye candy.

DIRECTOR: Michael Ninn, 1996, 106 min.

CAST: Ashlyn Gere, Annah Marie, Anna Malle, Jeanna Fine, Julie Rage, Kim Kitaine, Laura Palmer, P. J. Sparxx, Ruby, Victoria Paris, Vicca, John Decker, Hank Armstrong, Jeremy Steele, Mark Davis, Mike Horner, Peter North, Santino Lee, Tom Byron, Vince Voyeur

Dethroned

Miss New Hampshire was dethroned when it was discovered that she was an erotic dancer to get by while competing for the crown, and Thomas capitalizes on her story by creating this excellent docudrama starring the former Miss herself. The story is well embellished with plenty of sex and drama, and the Miss makes a great debut in her first adult performance.

DIRECTOR: Paul Thomas, 1999, 93 min.

CAST: Alex Taylor, Azlea, Corinne Williams, Inari Vachs, India, Johnni Black, Taylor St. Clair, Bill Williams, Bo, Jack Hammer, Peter Dawson, Randy Spears

Devil in Miss Jones 6

High-gloss and elaborate sets combine with lots of fetish costuming and obscure pop culture references to create a bizarre atmosphere of porn star sex and demons from hell on the loose. A woman opens a portal to hell (oops!) and two sex-crazed female demons emerge to have as much sex as possible and begin a reign of evil. Interesting visuals, though mostly lackluster sex.

DIRECTOR: Antonio Passolini, 1999, 130 min.

CAST: Juli Ashton, Vicca, Stacy Valentine, Tina Tyler, Nikkita, Peris Bleau, Lacey Ogden, Crystal Crawford, The Horny Little Man, John Strong, Randy Spears, Michael J. Coxx, Ian Daniels, J. J. Michaels

Dominant Women   Violet's Top Choice   Intense Chemistry   Extreme Sex Acts   Great for Newbies

The Dinner Party; Dinner Party 2: The Buffet

High production values grace both films, though more so in the first than the second, yet both share extremely hot sex and great camerawork. *Dinner Party* follows a group of guests through dinner as they confess their sexual fantasies and act on them, while #2 isn't a sequel but simply more great sexual fantasies and a climactic orgy.

The Dinner Party

DIRECTOR: Cameron Grant, 1994, 90 min.

CAST: Juli Ashton, Yvonne, Asia Carrera, Debi Diamond, Diva, Kaylan Nicole, Kylie Ireland, Crystal Gold, Vanessa Chase, Celeste, Tammi Parks, Norma Jeane, Catalina, Jewel Night, Daisy, Gerry Pike, Vince Vouyer, Marc Wallice, Frank Towers, Sean Michaels, Steve Drake, Randy West, Mark Davis

NOTE: Won several *AVN* awards in 1994.

Dinner Party 2: The Buffet

DIRECTOR: Seymore Butts, 1997, 100 min.

CAST: Stephanie Swift, Tyler Sweet, Nanna, Lisa Ann, Kimberly Kummings, Cortknee, Kelly Trump, Diamond, Mr. Marcus, Hakan Joel, Sean Michaels, Scott Styles, David Stone

Dinner Party at 6

A dramatic exploration of racism is the centerpiece for this nod to *Guess Who's Coming to Dinner,* with supercharged, passionate sex and terrific acting. A white woman and her black fiancé encounter a lot more than they expected from their friends and family on their wedding night dinner.

DIRECTOR: Sean Michaels, 1998, 93 min.

CAST: Naomi, Morgan Fairlane, Vanessa, Jacklyn Lick, Randy West, Mr. Marcus, Sean Michaels, Guy DiSilva, Chloe

NOTE: Won multiple *AVN* awards in 1998.

Woman Penetrates Man

Natural Cast

Unsightly Boob Job

Well-Made Film

Real Female Orgasm

Dog Walker

Although it's filled with raw and dirty sex, many people feel this to be one of John Leslie's great dramatic films, but I disagree. It's well shot and has a nice L.A. Mafia thread to the plot, but the disjointed story makes the sex seem out of place and the film plodding, though cerebral. You decide—it certainly won a lot of awards.

DIRECTOR: John Leslie, 1994, 110 min.

CAST: Lana Sands, Isis Nile, Krysti Lynn, Christina Angel, Michael Jones, Gerry Pike, Steven St. Croix, Jake Williams, Jamie Gillis, Tom Byron, Joey Silvera, Mark Davis, Alex Sanders, Jay Ashley

NOTE: Won several critics' choice awards.

(Jonathan Morgan's) Double Feature

Have you ever watched a monster movie and wanted to grab the camera, add a little *Son of Frankenstein* here, and a little *Monty Python* there, and make as many sex jokes as possible? The box cover fashions itself after old B-movie posters with an adult twist on the genre, claiming "Hear the moans of passion and the screams of terror!" and "Shot in shockingly-clear Vibe-O-Vision," and includes a comically frightened Serenity. Truth be told, it's just a taste of the two glorious B-movie spoofs inside, making for perhaps the smartest, funniest, mind-bogglingly dry-witted adult video ever made. It begins in black and white, introducing our hero (Randy Spears) and heroine (Serenity) in hilarious fake trailers, then leads us into separate features of frighteningly bad monster drama. The scenes invariably become sexual—how could they not with aliens from the planet Clitora, plus a detached penis from Abby Normal—and when they do, they're pretty dirty, and in color. Randy Spears is the Bruce Campbell of adult, and seeing him go over the top with these characters is worth the price of admission alone.

DIRECTOR: Jonathan Morgan, 1999, 114 min.

CAST: Serenity, Jewel De'Nyle, Randy Spears, Sana Fey, Mickey G, Shanna McCullough, Stephanie Swift, Herschel Savage

NOTE: Won several *AVN* awards in 1999.

Dominant Women   Violet's Top Choice   Intense Chemistry   Extreme Sex Acts   Great for Newbies

• •

Libido Films: Marianna Beck and Jeff Hafferkamp

WHEN *LIBIDO* MAGAZINE was in print, it was a quarterly journal of tasteful, all-orientation erotic photos, short stories, book and video reviews, and poetry. There was nothing like it, and today there still isn't, though *Libido* has found a home on the Web, where it also offers an independent line of adult features and educational films. Its budgets are low but the quality of the interaction between the nonadult industry cast members is very high. The plots are simple and realistic, focusing on fantasy realization within a heterosexual couple. The sex is nonformula, the bodies are all natural and tend to be tattooed, as the director usually uses contemporary Gen-X types, who seem to be experienced actors—though porn star Mickey G made an appearance in a (sadly) nonsex role in *Ecstatic Moments*. High chemistry, attention to character and motivation, great unconventional sex, and S/M mixed with sex are all great reasons to see *Libido*'s independent films. Check out *Thank You, Mistress; Sexual Ecstasy for Couples;* and *Urban Friction.*

• •

Dream Quest

Okay, so it's a fantasy film. Not just "porn fantasy" but like *Dungeons and Dragons* fantasy. Still, I have to admit, the budget and production values are amazingly high, high enough to make it seem like a Hollywood film—except that, like, all the women are big-boobed blondes and instead of telling "the gatekeeper" the really clever answer to a riddle in order to pass through the gate, they give him a blow job. Plot, schmot—it's got lots of porn stars and porn sex, with many fancy trimmings.

DIRECTOR: Brad Armstrong, 1999, 100 min.

CAST: Felecia, Asia Carrera, Sydnee Steele, Inari Vachs, Jessica Drake, Teri Starr, Amber Michaels, Bridgett Kerkove, Stephanie Swift, Jenna Jameson, Alexa Temtress, Randy Spears, Brad Armstrong, Dale DaBone, Anthony Crane, Herschel Savage, Devin Wolf, Evan Stone

NOTE: Has a spanking scene.

Woman Penetrates Man

Natural Cast

Unsightly Boob Job

Well-Made Film

Real Female Orgasm

Ecstatic Moments

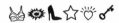

After lengthy introductions, three well-written and superbly performed vignettes explore three blistering sexual fantasies. In one, lesbian sex educator Tristan Taormino puts a male stud on a stage, puts him in his place, and uses him like a sex toy in front of a group of her peers, including Betty Dodson. In the second, famous sex writer Carol Queen is confronted by a sexy antiporn feminist, and Queen gives her a thorough (sexual) education. In the last, porn star Mickey G's powerful executive girlfriend gets the gift of her dreams—a night of S/M submission at the hands of an attractive couple. My only wish was that we got to see more of what Mickey G had to offer his girlfriend in the last scene.

DIRECTORS: Marianna Beck and Jack Hafferkamp, 1999, 78 min.

CAST: Gina Rome, Carol Queen, Tristan Taormino, Amy Jo Goddard, James Bonn, Mickey G, Claudio

NOTE: Independent filmmaker. S/M activities with sex.

Edge Play

The feature opens with an explosive female masturbation/female ejaculation onto the windshield of a parked, waiting limo in a dirty underground parking lot. And if that doesn't get your attention, the rest of the film will. A couple specializes in making the erotic fantasies of wealthy women come true, and the fantasies are intense, outrageous, and hot as hell. Legendary adult actress Marilyn Chambers stars as the woman who wants to try it, but isn't sure, and her confrontation of her own, nonpolitically-correct fantasies is fascinating.

DIRECTOR: Veronica Hart, 2001, 130 min.

CAST: Brooke Hunter, Marilyn Chambers, Chloe, Kimberly Chambers, Keisha, Kylie Ireland, Veronica Hart (nonsex), Anthony Crane (nonsex), Bruno Assix, Dale DaBone, Don Hollywood, Eric Masterson, George Kaplan (nonsex), Jay Ashley, Jamie Gillis, Joel Lawrence, Kyle Stone, Marty Romano, Nick Manning, Randy Spears, Tyce Bune, Valentino

NOTE: Contains a female ejaculation scene.

Dominant Women

Violet's Top Choice

Intense Chemistry

Extreme Sex Acts

Great for Newbies

Euphoria

This film took home awards in nine categories, with incredible cinematography, a complex and highly intelligent plot, fantastic acting, and out-of-this-world production values. In an apocalyptic future, the populace is controlled through their personal spending and debt, and once you go into debt, you become property of the State. One option to escape the institutionalized slavery is to become a test subject for the mind-control sex drug U4. Sydnee Steele shines as the willful, impossible-to-break test subject, as does Ava Vincent as the ruthless government puppet. Wow.

DIRECTOR: Brad Armstrong, 2001, 90 min.

CAST: Sydnee Steele, Devinn Lane, Inari Vachs, Asia Carrera, Bridgette Kerkove, Ava Vincent, Felecia, Jezebelle Bond, Nikita Denise, Shay Sweet, Charlene Aspen, Tanya Danielle, April, Lee Stone, Dillion Day, Mike Horner, Cheyne Collins, Billy Glide, Pat Myne, Evan Stone, Mark Davis, Erik Everhard, Nick Manning, Dale DaBone

NOTE: Won nine *AVN* awards.

Every Woman Has a Fantasy 3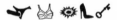

More frustrated wives, but this time it's the talented and sexually authentic Juli Ashton in the lead role as a wife who works in a sex club to let off steam. An oft-recommended favorite by women-owned sex shops, it contains oodles of fantasies including exhibitionism, orgies, toys, and voyeurism, all from a female perspective.

DIRECTOR: Edwin Durrell, 1995, 100 min.

CAST: Melissa Hill, Juli Ashton, Kia, Felecia, Ariana, Rebecca Bardoux, Alec Metro, Steve Drake, Peter North, Mark Davis

Woman Penetrates Man

Natural Cast

Unsightly Boob Job

Well-Made Film

Real Female Orgasm

Exstasy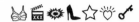

The acting, complex story line, sexual chemistry, and direction of this 35mm film earn high ratings. Tyffany Million (known for her onscreen sexual aggressiveness) desperately hopes marriage will straighten up her life, even though she can't seem to leave behind her promiscuous habits. She leads a double life, encourageed by the lickable British actress Sarah Jane Hamilton in her adventures in an underground sex club. Hamilton is notable in any movie; with her genuine arousal, normal, squishy body, and gushing orgasms she never fails to steal the show. Meanwhile, the sleazy loser Million's husband hires to uncover her secret sets out to steal her for himself. Shot entirely on location in San Francisco and New Orleans. More Robert McCallum films are in Chapter 7, "The Classics: Porn's Golden Age."

DIRECTOR: Robert McCallum, 1995, 103 min.

CAST: Sarah Jane Hamilton, Tyffany Million, Tom Byron, Steve Drake

Eyes of Desire

A woman peeps at her neighbors through a telescope and gets an eyeful, as does the man spying on her, and he'll do anything to have her. The pacing lags, but the female perspective and absence of formulaic sex are notable.

DIRECTOR: Candida Royalle, 1998, 95 min.

CAST: Jenteal, Sharon Mitchell, Missy, Herschel Savage, Tom Byron, Tony Tedeschi, Mickey G, Chloe

NOTE: No anal, a cross-dressing man, plus a scene with former real-life husband and wife Missy and Mickey G

Eyes of Desire 2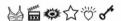

The voyeurs return, this time with the man seducing the woman into trying a number of new sexual experiences, much like *9 ½ Weeks*. The pacing lags, but the fantasies are great. In one scene, the lead character picks up a rough mechanic and has sex with him front of her window so that her male voyeur can watch.

DIRECTOR: Candida Royalle, 1999, 71 min.

CAST: Jeannie Pepper, Missy, Lexington Steele, Mickey G, Ramon Fernandez, Steve Drake

NOTE: Internal ejaculation; the lead characters were husband and wife in real life; and the first anal sex scene in a Royalle film (Missy).

Dominant Women	Violet's Top Choice	Intense Chemistry	Extreme Sex Acts	Great for Newbies

Façade

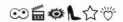

This tense drama packs in more intense sex scenes on one tape than most other adult films, and has an all-star cast to boot. Randy Spears is a man whose wife openly cheats on him, and their relationship is a ticking time bomb of sexual revenge that explodes on a weekend when she pushes the sexual antics to the boiling point when a group of friends come over and the party gets out of hand. Each sex scene simmers with emotional tension, and one of the film's climaxes happens when Spears enacts his first infidelity. This film is top-rate in every category, and though the story is dark, the sex fits in perfectly with the script, character motivation, and story—a rare quality in porn features.

DIRECTOR: Paul Thomas, 2000, 100 min.

CAST: Kira Kener, Inari Vachs, April, Sydnee Steele, Bobby Vitale, Vince Voyeur, Eric Everhard

NOTE: Multiple *AVN* award winner in 2000.

Face Dance

John "Buttman" Stagliano's first full-length feature film is an epic, combining his then-obsession for the erotic immediacy of sexual contact with the face—facial come shots, smothering, and so on. Rocco Siffredi comes to Hollywood as an Italian movie stud, whose pressures on the set conspire with his repressed sexual fixations and reduce him to a man helplessly in thrall to his sexual obsessions. Note the riveting scene in which Tina Tyler puts Siffredi in his place.

DIRECTOR: John Stagliano, 1993; 2 tapes/discs, 120 min. each

CAST, PART 1: Tina Tyler, Sierra, Chrissy Ann, Roscoe Bowltree, Rebecca Bardoux, Francesca Le, Sheila Stone, Britany O'Connell, Tiffany Million, Cody O'Connor, Angel Ash, Tiffany Mynx, Kiss, Kris Newz, Tom Byron, Joey Silvera, Steve Drake, John Stagliano, Randy Spears, Toni Tedeschi, Rick Smears, Brockton O'Toole, Woody Long

CAST, PART 2: Tiffany Mynx, Tina Tyler, Sierra, Chrissy Ann, Rebecca Bardoux, Francesca Le, Sheila Stone, Kiss, Brittany O'Connell, Tiffany Million, Cody O'Connor, Angel Ash, Toni Tedeschi, Tom Byron, Joey Silvera, Steve Drake, John Stagliano, Rocco Siffredi, Kris Newz

NOTE: Won five *AVN* and *Adam Film World* awards.

Woman Penetrates Man

Natural Cast

Unsightly Boob Job

Well-Made Film

Real Female Orgasm

Fade to Black

This fantastic, dark drama begins by introducing us to three amateur porn film-makers who want to make it big: a director, his cameraman, and the female talent (the director's girlfriend). They go to L.A. to meet the director's hero (a big-time porn producer), and in no time the wanna-be director is reduced to a suitcase pimp, while all three of them are turned against one another through their own selfish motives. The plot twists one more murderous time, and if the plot doesn't keep you busy, the terrific, emotionally driven sex will. A fantastic film in every category.

DIRECTOR: Paul Thomas, 2001, 130 min.

CAST: Julie Meadows, Taylor St. Clair, Taylor Hayes, Adajja, Rikki Lixxx, Meriesa Arroyo, Tony Tedeschi, Dale DaBone, Jason McCain, Eric Everhard, Joey Ray, Voodoo, Mark Wood

NOTE: Swept the 2002 AVN awards, taking five honors.

Fade to Blue

The minimal plot centers on Juli Ashton returning home to contemplate her past sexual memories, almost making this an all-sex feature, but with a high budget and lush, slow-mo visuals.

DIRECTOR: Michael Ninn, 1997, 118 min.

CAST: Vicca, Amber Lynn, Nikita, Juli Ashton, Asia Carrera, Houston, Earl Slate, James Bonn, Mr. Marcus, Colt Steele, Alec Metro, Mark Davis

Dominant Women　　　Violet's Top Choice　　　Intense Chemistry　　　Extreme Sex Acts　　　Great for Newbies

The Fashionistas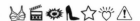

In another stunning epic by Stagliano (and possibly Buttman's finest film ever), Rocco plays a famous Italian fashion designer who comes to L.A. to find a designer for his new fetishwear line, much to the chagrin of his bitchy line buyer. He's seduced by some extremely clever pranks and public stunts masterminded by rogue fetish designers, The Fashionistas. But that's not all, and while the story twists and turns around the head Fashionistas designer's plot to draw the S/M-curious Rocco into her BDSM underground, the otherworldly, heart-pounding S/M sex punctuates the story line. Unbelievable production values and acting, with unnervingly rough and nonstop sex. Clamps, clips, whips, chains, extreme penetrations, suffocation, spitting, ponygirls, unenhanced female bodies, and more make this film as intense as it is realistic. Not for the novice porn viewer.

DIRECTOR: John "Buttman" Stagliano, 2002, 280 min.

CAST: Belladonna, Careena Collins (nonsex), Chelsea Blue, Caroline Pierce, Friday, Gia, Kate Frost, Monique, Ruby Richards (nonsex), Sharon Wild, Tricia Devereaux (nonsex), Taylor St. Clair, Billy Glyde, Brandon Iron, Kane, Mark Ashley, Manuel Ferrara, Rocco Siffredi

NOTE: S/M activities with sex. Won an unprecedented ten *AVN* awards in 2003.

Flamenco Ecstasy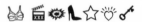

Legendary European cult director Joe D'Amato turned in a number of excellent porn films before he died, and this is a great example of mature Spanish porn. A stunningly beautiful Spanish woman will do anything to seduce the only man she's ever loved—a matador. This character-driven plot weaves sex seamlessly into each fully dimensional character's pathos.

DIRECTOR: Joe D'Amato, 1997, 70 min.

CAST: Maria De Sanchez, Jessica Lange, Heros, Elisabeth King, Monica Orsini, Hakan Joel, Steve Drake, Oliver Sanchez, Jolt Gabor, Mike DeVinci

NOTE: Foreign release. Contains a graphic bullfight, may have bad dubbing.

Woman Penetrates Man	Natural Cast	Unsightly Boob Job	Well-Made Film	Real Female Orgasm

Flashpoint

Like firemen? How about firewomen? A female firefighter searches for love in this compelling drama that has authentic sets and sizzling sex. Good introduction to Jenna Jameson.

DIRECTOR: Brad Armstrong, 1997, 120 min.

CAST: Jenna Jameson, Sindee Coxx, Jill Kelly, Asia Carrera, Brittany Andrews, Veronica Hart (nonsex), Missy, Jonathan Morgan, TT Boy, Steve Drake, Brad Armstrong, Mickey G, Johnni Black, Sydnee Steele

NOTE: Won multiple *AVN* awards in 1994.

Forever Night

In this complex tale of living purgatory, a man can only watch but not participate in the sex staged for his torture. The sex is intense and raw, the visuals are stunning, and the frustrated man dishes out nasty, dirty talk (with help from Jeanna Fine) to punctuate the film.

DIRECTOR: Michael Ninn, 1997, 87 min.

CAST: Jill Kelly, Stacy Valentine, Jeanna Fine, Liza Harper, Brooke Lane, Raylene, Britany Andrews, Robert Rose, Jamie Gillis, Earl Slate, Peter Romero, John Decker, Colt Steele

The Gift

Romantic and achingly sweet, this tale follows a blanket imbued with an experience of romantic longing that prompts everyone who comes in contact with it to consummate their most heartfelt sexual impulses. Sensuous lovemaking is the theme here.

DIRECTOR: Candida Royalle, 1997, 87 min.

CAST: Shanna McCullough, Mark Davis, Micky Lynn, Diane Cannon, David Wells, Angel Smith, Eric Jeter, Joey D.

NOTE: No anal.

| Dominant Women | Violet's Top Choice | Intense Chemistry | Extreme Sex Acts | Great for Newbies |

Ginger Lynn Is Torn

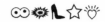

A world-famous soap star, Ginger Lynn, who is lonely and horny as hell, fantasizes about being passed around by three guys, screwed by Juli Ashton with a strap-on, and going down on an anonymous man (Sean Michaels). She visits some old pals, most notably also-horny, sexy old pals Chloe, Devin Wolf, and John Decker. She eventually finds herself in super-hot trysts with each of them (including a satisfying girl–girl with Chloe and an amazing blow job with Wolf). Then she's torn—whom will she choose? Who cares! The plot isn't very exciting, but there are ten sex scenes and they're all good.

DIRECTOR: Veronica Hart, 1999, 145 min.

CAST: Jenteal, Juli Ashton, Stacy Valentine, Tina Tyler, Kylie Ireland, Ginger Lynn, Mia Smiles, Rayveness, Julian, Devin Wolf, Michael J. Coxx, Alec Metro, Sean Michaels, John Decker

Hamlet

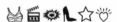

No expense was spared in the making of this raunchy European version of Hamlet, including on-location shooting in a castle, incredible costumes, and more than fifty attractive cast members. Decadence of the royals at its finest. Find more Joe D'Amato films in Chapter 7, "The Classics: Porn's Golden Age."

DIRECTOR: Joe D'Amato, 1996, 76 min.

CAST: Christoph Clark, Sarah Young, Richard Langin, Roberto Malone, Maeva, Vicky, Tanya LaRiviere, Joe D'Amato, Carol Nash, Valentina Martinez, Shalimar, In-X-Cess

NOTE: Foreign release.

Hayseed

It's a country-bumpkin comedy of errors, where Chloe runs around looking sexy in coveralls and fingering much more than her shotgun. Dense as her "lucky melon," Bobbi Jo decides to leave the farm and go to Hollywood, where she ends up in the seedy adult industry, meanwhile leaving behind horny-as-a-bunny Chloe, dumb-as-a-doorstop Evan Stone, and conniving pie-baker Julie Meadows. If this sounds silly, it is, but it's a whole lotta bad-pun, dry-humor fun with terrific sex.

DIRECTOR: Chloe, 2002, 98 min.

CAST: Chloe, Julie Meadows, Justine Romee, Kylie Ireland, Nina Hartley, Zana, Evan Stone, Joel Lawrence, Kyle Stone, Nikko Knight, Pat Myne

Woman Penetrates Man	Natural Cast	Unsightly Boob Job	Well-Made Film	Real Female Orgasm

Heart Strings

The trials and tribulations of an L.A. rock band fuel this character-driven drama, where sex with bandmates is the wedge threatening to force apart musicians on the verge of success. The sex scenes are key to the plot, and it's refreshing to see a film whose plot doesn't stop for the obligatory sex scene—plus the sex is excellent. What's more, the porn stars playing the musicians are really musicians, and every acting effort is utterly beleivable. Although it's not lavishly filmed, the video excels in practically every other category.

DIRECTOR: Chloe, 2002, 103 min.

CAST: Aria, Chloe, Daisy Chain, Kylie Ireland, Wendy Divine, Eric Masterson, Kyle Stone, Steve Hatcher, Tyler Wood

The Hottest Bid

Couple Jessica and Marty are suffering from middle-age frustration, and for swingin' kicks they attend a bachelor charity auction where women bid against one another for a date with a sexy guy. One of Jessica's pals gets Marty, and Jessica gets a guy with a big dog. Marty gets a night being tutored in light BDSM with some Tantric sex, and Jessica gets an anticlimactic picnic followed by some romance in a cabin. Nice, light, soft-core romantic fare.

DIRECTOR: Deborah Shames, 1995, 90 min.

CAST: Lenore Andriel, Gwen Somers, Belinda Farrell, Tracy Miller, Dennis Matthews

NOTE: Soft core, no explicit sex or genital close-ups.

I Dream of Jenna

Like it's namesake, the film features Jenna Jameson as the genie in a bottle that grants wishes. The whole film has a lighthearted, fun approach and packs in ten sex scenes, including a scene with Jenna and her real-life husband, director Justin Sterling. High budgets and an enthusiastic cast.

DIRECTor: Justin Sterling, 2002, 120 min.

CAST: Jenna Jameson, Nikita Denise, Autumn, Jewel De'Nyle, Aurora Snow, Lezley Zen, Brittany Andrews, Flick Shagwell, Karianna, Inari Vachs, Steven St. Croix, Randy Spears, Jay Ashley, Eric Everhard

NOTE: Won an *AVN* award for the girl–girl scene.

Dominant Women	Violet's Top Choice	Intense Chemistry	Extreme Sex Acts	Great for Newbies

Immortal

An all-star, all-über-babe cast carries off this soft, romantic tale of the Greek Goddess of Music (a beautiful Jill Kelly), who inspires men and then leaves them—that is, until she falls in love with one man and must choose between her immortality and true love. Great acting and sexual performances, especially when the goddesses come after her and rain sexual terror—and pleasure—on hapless men and excited women alike. High production values, with a slightly soft-focus feel in the romantic scenes.

DIRECTOR: Michael Raven, 2001, 95 min.

CAST: Tabitha Stevens, Dee, Haven, Devon, Asia Carrera, Tawny Roberts, Shayla LaVeaux, Monica Sweetheart, Jill Kelly

Jekyll and Hyde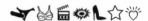

The costumes and setting are fantastic, with loads of Victorian dresses and corsets, and filmed entirely on location in Budapest. The best part about the location is that the majority of the cast is European, meaning there are all kinds of beautiful natural bodies (in fact only the lead, Taylor Hayes, has a tit job), decent acting, and a lot of great fucking. The story line is what you'd expect from the title— Taylor returns from a girls' school to find her mansion deserted, her daddy missing, and only his faithful manservant remaining. She spends time in Dad's lab, eventually uncovering the serum he developed and trying it out on herself, only to become an evil sex maniac (like he did before he went AWOL). We get to see both his murderous exploits in tantalizing detail and Taylor's erotic descent into madness in carefully layered storytelling scenes. There are all sorts of great scenarios such as (my favorite) an encounter where Taylor punishes a man for keeping information from her about her dad (and he ends up with a lashing and a lit candle up his behind), plus repeat scenes of a bordello I wish really existed. There are a few misses, but they're really two minor continuity flaws and I can see why they were left in—the scenes were really working, and that says it all for the film. This is great porn.

DIRECTOR: Paul Thomas, 2000, 93 min.

CAST: Alette, Daniella, Fernanda, Genevive, Judyh, Kate More, Taylor Hayes, Alberto Rey, Bobby Vitale, Frank Gun, Frank Major, Ian Daniels, John Kossa, Julian, Kallinger Horst, Leslie Taylor, Mike Foster

NOTE: Has a bloody murder scene.

| Woman Penetrates Man | Natural Cast | Unsightly Boob Job | Well-Made Film | Real Female Orgasm |

Justine: Nothing to Hide 2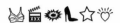

Roxanne Blaze is an incredible, fresh-faced actress who delivers lines that are searing, and is one of the most insatiable women to grace the blue screen. In Thomas's masterpiece, she turns in a performance so strong you'll be transfixed and have to watch the film to its powerful climax. A young female writer is covering a story about sex toy shops while her boyfriend is out of town, and unwittingly begins a torrid affair with his father.

DIRECTOR: Paul Thomas, 1994, 90 min.

CAST: Dyanna Lauren, Roxanne Blaze, Leanna Foxxx, Tianna, Alex Sanders, Brad Armstrong, Paul Thomas (nonsex), Mike Horner, Nick East (nonsex)

NOTE: Won eight *AVN* awards, no safer sex, contains a mullet.

Latex

This film put Ninn on the map and took the 1996 *AVN* awards by storm as an unsuspecting porn audience was treated to stunning visuals, excellent cinematography, lots of L.A.-style industrial atmosphere, fetish clothes, and strong chemistry between performers. The sci-fi story revolves around a man who is tormented by psychic visions of other people's sexual fantasies.

DIRECTOR: Michael Ninn, 1995, 120 min.

CAST: Juli Ashton, Jeanna Fine, Jordan Lee, Sunset Thomas, Tyffany Million, Debi Diamond, Leanna Foxxx, Veronica Hart (nonsex), Barbara Doll, Emerald Estrada, Tasha Blades, Kelly Nichols, Zach Adams, Colt Steel, Bricks Majors, Vince Voyeur, Ritchie Razor, Cal Jammer, Jonathan Morgan, Tom Byron, Mark Davis

Note: Won multiple *AVN* awards in 1995.

| Dominant Women | Violet's Top Choice | Intense Chemistry | Extreme Sex Acts | Great for Newbies |

Les Vampyres

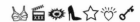

Although it's somewhat cheesily marketed with a companion comic book, the movie itself is a visual delight. Heavy in contrast lighting, great costumes, and fabulous sets, it reminds me of the late 1960s and 1970s lesbian vampire films in both scenery and content. In it, a trio of timeless vamps is leisurely feeding and killing their way down the Pacific Coast Highway, and take a rest in a B & B in Big Sur. There, a "nice" couple is checking in for a romantic weekend away, and sparks fly in the foyer when the queen vampire makes eye contact with the girlfriend. Her fate is sealed, and so, it seems, is her boyfriend's. The plot is akin to the terrific cult lesbian vampire film *The Velvet Vampire* (head lesbian vampire steals girlfriend, bad news for boyfriend) and to Jess Franco's *Bare Breasted Countess* (killing is done after the sex act: the blood is drunk from the male genitals). The blood-drinking scenes are messy and vivid, and the sex scenes are, too, especially since the actresses are heavily Goth-styled. Fantastic acting, great sex without typical porn lighting and gyno-close-ups, and real passion between the actors.

DIRECTOR: James Avalon, 2000, 87 min.

CAST: Ava Vincent, Samantha, Syren, Violet Love, Wendi Knight, Brandon Iron, Brick Majors, Jack Hammer, Joel Lawrence, Nick Orleans (nonsex)

NOTE: Won three *AVN* awards; scenes of blood and violence.

Les Vampyres 2

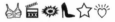

Not a sequel as much as a beautiful and sophisticated continuation of the theme. Female vamp Lilliana is after the lesbian vampire who killed her man several centuries ago, and Lilliana will stop at nothing to trap and kill her in revenge. The lighting and costumes add to the atmosphere in every scene, most notably the ethereal couples partner swap that closely echoes the cult film *The Hunger*—and won an *AVN* award. A very high quality, complete film with sex that makes sense in the script, sensual and erotic filming of the sex scenes, and talented actors.

DIRECTOR: James Avalon, 2002, 99 min.

CAST: Gina Ryder, Holly Hollywood, Ava Vincent, Kate Frost, Katja Kean, Kelli Sparks, Misty Rain, Nikita Denise, Syren, Wendi Knight, John Decker, Hammer, Joel Lawrence, Marc Davis, Nick East, Nick Orleans (nonsex)

NOTE: Won an *AVN* award, scenes of blood and violence, a scene with then-couple Ava Vincent and John Decker.

Woman Penetrates Man

Natural Cast

Unsightly Boob Job

Well-Made Film

Real Female Orgasm

Lisa

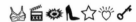

Stunningly beautiful, Lisa is a French girl who starts out the film in a heated tryst with her lame boyfriend and his pal, only to realize what a loser her boyfriend is for treating her badly, so she sets out on her own sexual quest across the roads of America. An enjoyable character-driven story that has lots of genuine, passionate sex and great cinematography.

DIRECTOR: Kris Kramski, 2000, 1997

CAST: Cassidy, Houston, Lisa Harper, Tatianna, Alec Metro, Jeremy Steele, Michael J. Cox

Looking In

If you want a film that looks and feels like a real movie, but with lots of explicit sex woven into the plot, this Paul Thomas epic should be at the top of your list. Creepy, moody, expertly filmed in natural light, and with subtle use of wide-angle shots for narrative transition, it's a compelling film from start to finish. An attractive nonporn couple moves into their dream home and discover that things are not what they seem when their neighbors begin to engage in increasingly unusual sex acts. Fantastic exploration of sex and emotion, voyeurism and infidelity by a stunning cast who can act as passionate as they fuck—no easy feat in this genre. Director Paul Thomas weaves sex with the plot perfectly, to create a perfect adult film. Oh, and the kinky hot-wax scene will definitely leave some viewers breathless.

DIRECTOR: Paul Thomas, 2002, 108 min.

CAST: Savanna Samson, Dale Dabone, Taylor St. Claire, Mickey G, Ann Marie, Steven St. Croix, Dru Berrymore

Love's Passion

A romance novelist writes her own story of lost love and the wish for redemption into the Civil War–era piece she's working on, and the result is her story being told in overlapping time frames. A period piece mixed with modern human drama, as romantic and yearning as it is packed with sensuous, tender, and raw sex. Period sex scene is slightly marred by actor's tattoos.

DIRECTOR: Veronica Hart, 1998, 120 min.

CAST: Nikita, Juli Ashton, Tina Tyler, Rayveness, Shayla LaVeaux, Herschel Savage, Tyce Bune, Colt Steele, John Decker, Mickey G

NOTE: Internal ejaculation; shot on film.

| Dominant Women | Violet's Top Choice | Intense Chemistry | Extreme Sex Acts | Great for Newbies |

The Marquis De Sade
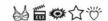

This high-budget Italian sex blockbuster builds character and tension between Rocco and Rosa Carciolla, while loosely following the tale of master pervert De Sade. Great acting, sets, and costumes play second fiddle to the intense sex scenes.

DIRECTOR: Joe D'Amato, 1995, 85 min.

CAST: Allona, Marie, Mark, Mike Foster, Rocco Siffredi, Rosa Caracciolo, Shalimar, Valentina, Vicky

NOTE: S/M activities with sex. Foreign release. Won an *AVN* award in 1995.

The Masseuse
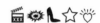

In a noir drama worthy of a regular feature film, Randy Spears plays a naïve man who visits a self-destructive sex worker—a masseuse—and winds up becoming obsessed with her. Excellent performances from the actors all around. The entire film is full of terrific sex, including authentic female orgasms.

DIRECTOR: Paul Thomas, 1990, 85 min.

CAST: Danielle Rodgers (nonsex), Hyapatia Lee, Porsche Lynn (nonsex), Viper (nonsex), Paul Thomas (nonsex), Randy Spears

Masseuse 2

Not a sequel to *Masseuse* but a continuation of its theme. Ashlyn Gere delivers an incredible performance as a masseuse who interprets her job as an art form. But she takes it too far, and while she (and her coworkers) deliver amazingly concentrated sex scenes, her personal "mission" drives her over the edge and into violent, self-destructive oblivion. Dark, tense, and dramatic, with a surprising script.

DIRECTOR: Paul Thomas, 1994, 120 min.

CAST: Ashlyn Gere, Asia Carrera, Kristina West, Carl Radford, Tony Tedeschi, Steven St. Croix

Woman Penetrates Man   Natural Cast   Unsightly Boob Job   Well-Made Film   Real Female Orgasm

Masseuse 3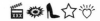

More terrific acting and taut sexual encounters in this continuation of the sex worker/obsession theme. An awkward young man loses his virginity to an uncaring, very sexually active college girl, and sees a masseuse with a "heart of gold" as a vessel for his unfulfilled desires. While he pines for the college girl, the masseuse breaks her rules of falling for her client, and none of the misguided characters find easy answers.

DIRECTOR: Paul Thomas, 1998, 120 min.

CAST: Lexi Eriksson, Tina Tyler, Sharon Mitchell, Katie Gold, Nancy Vee, Melissa Hill, Leanni Lei, Tia Bella, Chloe Nicole, Taylor Hayes, Jamie Gillis, Herschel Savage, Mr. Marcus, James Bonn

Michael Ninn's Perfect

In what may be Ninn's most exquisite piece of visual porn art to date, like the title says, everything in this lavishly produced film is perfect. Each shot is meticulously staged, lighting is crisp, the flow of scenes is seamless, and the performers themselves are the epitome of seamless, visually "perfected" porn stars. The cinematography is stunning, and it's really cool to see the "bullet time" method of filming (where time slows and the camera view rotates to another perspective) used in an adult film, which is really what we were all thinking of when we first saw *The Matrix*. Slick and sophisticated, the film follows the theme of *Blade Runner,* where future cop Nick Manning is assigned the task of hunting and eliminating four hypersexual androids disguised as humans. Plenty of anal sex, DPs, and the usual formula sex looks a thousand times more interesting in this sleek production, and much of the all-star cast put energy and fire into their encounters. And if the boot-licking scene with Tina Tyler doesn't grab your attention, check your pulse.

DIRECTOR: Michael Ninn, 2002, 129 min.

CAST: Brooke Hunter, Dru Berrymore, Flick Shagwell, Fujiko Kano, Jodie Moore, Julia Ann, Kelly Steele, Kiwi, Kristal Summers, Layla-Jade, Mia Smiles, Monica Mayhem, Nikita Denise, Sabrine Maui, Shay Sights, Tina Tyler, Wendy Divine, Art Core, Dale DaBone, Don Hollywood, Eric Masterson, Hamilton Steele, Nick Manning, Tyce Bune

Dominant Women

Violet's Top Choice

Intense Chemistry

Extreme Sex Acts

Great for Newbies

Michael Ninn's Ritual

As with many Ninn features, main character Vicca is insane (or is she?) and is in sexual torment, being led through each of her sexual fantasies (or are they experiences)? Lots of fetish gear and fetish acts round out the sex, including a medical scene, industrial scenery, and bizarre, dream-like sequences.

DIRECTOR: Michael Ninn, 1998, 100 min.

CAST: Nikita, Vicca, Danielle Rogers, Dee, Katja Kean, Julian, Keri Windsor, Jenny MacArthur, Tyce Bune, Damien Wolf, Randy Spears, Evan Stone, James Bonn, Eric Price

Mobster's Wife

In a cleverly constructed, humorous story of deceit and the perils of spreading yourself too thin, a mobster on the lam must remain in hiding yet maintain his three girlfriends and meet their ever-increasing and ridiculous sexual demands—his girlfriends being his wife, mistress, and rival mobster's (adult) daughter.

DIRECTOR: Paul Thomas, 1998, 120 min.

CAST: Stephanie Swift, Kelly Jean, Katie Gold, Shay Sweet, Sommer Daze, Derrick Lane, Mr. Marcus, Vince Voyeur

My Surrender

This romantic, heartache-saturated flick centers on a woman who films couples having sex, but is so wrapped up in her own fear of intimacy that she's all alone. A mysterious, mullet-headed stranger comes into her life, determined to break through the ice, despite his dorky haircut. The title suggests that she surrenders, but it's a little more complicated than that, and is actually a pretty good film.

DIRECTOR: Candida Royalle, 1996, 82 min.

CAST: Jenna Fine, Jill Kelly, Nici Sterling, April Hunter, Robert Landon, Alex Sanders, Mark Davis

NOTE: Contains a mullet, scenes feature two real-life porn couples; no facials, no anal.

Woman Penetrates Man

Natural Cast

Unsightly Boob Job

Well-Made Film

Real Female Orgasm

One Size Fits All

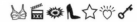

This film is a fun, lighthearted tale about a magical dress that, once it's on, makes the wearer aroused and irresistible to any man (though in this film the dress is only ever tested by heterosexual women, so we may never know its full potential). Discovered by accident while a woman is shopping—she has a steamy tryst in the dressing room—the dress is taken home and quickly becomes hot property among her gal-pals once they figure it out. Excellent film with heated, genuine sex.

DIRECTOR: Candida Royalle, 1998, 79 min.

CAST: Nina Hartley, Melissa Hill, Missy, Gina Rome, Candida Royalle, Peter Romera, Alex Sanders, Tom Byron

NOTE: Internal ejaculation, no anal.

The Operation

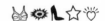

Although difficult to find, this is one of the most erotic, unusual, and important short adult films made to date. Winner at the New York Underground Film Festival, this explicit, futuristic film is shot entirely in infrared, a process in which anything hot shows up as white, while cold shows up as black, making it an amazing black-and-white film. Gorgeous Gina Velour is a doctor whose treatment for her male patient is sex in the operating theater. Trails of saliva turn black in the cold air, while arousal turns body parts white hot—the result is a startling aphrodisiac.

DIRECTOR: Jacob Pander, 1996, 13 min.

CAST: Gina Velour, Otto Wreck

NOTE: Independent filmmaker.

Pornogothic

This B-movie female vampire film stars a bevy of beauties and has a decent plot, but just doesn't quite pull off enough authenticity to rise above the medium production values and the mostly mediocre sex (a couple of exceptions being Brad Armstrong and Asia Carrera's scenes). A group of female vampires is roaming the streets, introducing hapless men to the food chain, so detective Armstrong, with his own complicated relationship problems clouding his judgment, is called on the case.

DIRECTOR: Jonathan Morgan, 1998, 115 min.

CAST: Stephanie Swift, Katie Gold, Missy, Serenity, Asia Carrera, Azlea Antistia, Ian Daniels, Dave Cummings, Mickey G, Alex Sanders, Brad Armstrong

Dominant Women

Violet's Top Choice

Intense Chemistry

Extreme Sex Acts

Great for Newbies

Psycho Sexuals; Psycho Sexuals 2

All there is to the plot is the theme of early conceptions of virtual reality, which is the excuse for aggressive women to have sex—often group sex—with anonymous men.

Psycho Sexuals

DIRECTOR: Gregory Dark (the Dark Bros.), 1997, 104 min.

CAST: Chloe, Leanna Heart, Missy, Nikita, Ruby, Sid Deuce, Taren Steele, Guy DaSilva, Jeremy Steele, Mickey G, Michael J. Cox, Paul Cox, Sean Rider, Tommy Gunn, Vince Voyeur

NOTE: Contains a female ejaculation scene.

Psycho Sexuals 2

DIRECTOR: Gregory Dark (the Dark Bros.), 1998, 120 min.

CAST: Alexandra Nice, Shayla LaVeaux, India, Solveigh, Jamaica, Pat Myne, Roberto Malone, Rod Fontana

Revelations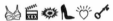

Set in the future, when sexual enjoyment is forbidden, a woman discovers video-tapes that contain explicit scenes of couples having sizzling sex and that awaken her to a whole new reality. This was Royalle's first solid directorial effort, and the continuity, editing, overall quality, and concentrated characters show it. Three great sex scenes focus on the women getting off, and overall it seems more an R-rated film with sex than a porn film (no genital close-ups).

DIRECTOR: Candida Royalle, 1992, 120 min.

CAST: Amy Rapp, Ava Grace, Michele Capozzi, Nicole London, Paris Phillips, Colin Matthews, Martin London

NOTE: No facials, no anal, no close–ups.

Woman Penetrates Man

Natural Cast

Unsightly Boob Job

Well-Made Film

Real Female Orgasm

Sex; Sex 2: Fate

With a nod to the theme of *La Dolce Vita*, these films center on the empty world of celebrity life and the yearning for something more. Dark and neo-noir, both films show the betrayal and deceit behind the glossy world of entertainment, blending eloquent, stylized sex scenes and attractive actors with the emptiness of the characters' lives.

Sex

DIRECTOR: Michael Ninn, 1993.

CAST: Sunset Thomas, Tyffany Million, Gerry Pike, Chasey Lain, Jon Dough, Debi Diamond, Misty Rain, Diva, Diedre Holland, Asia Carrera

Sex 2

DIRECTOR: Michael Ninn, 1994, 85 min.

CAST: Christy Canyon, Crystal Wilder, Nikki Dial, P. J. Sparxx, Max Hardcore (nonsex), Mike Horner, Rocco Siffredi, Tom Byron, Terry Thomas

The Shipwreck

Filmed entirely on location in Hawaii and predating *Survivor* by a few years, this tight and tense film focuses on plot and character, though it has some slow pacing issues in the beginning. But once it gets started you'll want to find out what happens to the eight castaways shipwrecked on an island, who find that sex becomes the currency for power, food, and safety.

DIRECTOR: Paul Thomas, 1998, 90 min.

CAST: Stephanie Swift, Missy, Deva Station, Mickey G, Marc Wallice

Dominant Women

Violet's Top Choice

Intense Chemistry

Extreme Sex Acts

Great for Newbies

Shock

In a sequel to his film *Latex,* Ninn delivers more of the same liquid gothic visuals and constant sex from rapacious performers draped in fetish wear, as they torment their captive viewer—which is actually *you.* The scenes ooze fetish, and some of the activities cater or allude to fetish or S/M practices, though no actual S/M is in any of the scenes.

DIRECTOR: Michael Ninn, 1996, 120 min.

CAST: Jeanna Fine, Sharon Kane, Juli Ashton, Kia, Jill Kelly, Felecia, Sunset Thomas, Tyffany Million, Tricia Yen, Caressa Savage, Jenny Blair, Ona Zee (nonsex), Misty Rain, Rebecca Lord, Marine Cartier, John Decker, Peter North, Mark Davis, Sean Rider, Vince Voyeur, TT Boy

NOTE: Won multiple *AVN* awards in 1996, including Best Outrageous Sex Scene.

Show and Tell

In a "reality-TV" documentary approach, director Thomas interviews Kobe Tai, Stephanie Swift, Juli Rage, and Lexi Leigh about their work—sex. In what resemble four short "Deep Insides," each woman talks about her sexual fantasies, strips in a one-on-one with the camera, and has sex with a medley of partners and sex toys.

DIRECTOR: Paul Thomas, 1998, 105 min.

Cast: Kobe Tai, Stephanie Swift, Lexi Leigh, Julie Rage, Sindee Coxx, Krista Maze, Gina Rome, TT Boy, Claudio, Tommy Gunn, Alex Sanders, Byron Long

Sinful Rella

Julie Meadows plays the eponymous role of the downtrodden scullery maid, and though there is only one evil stepsister, she and the evil mother pack in enough sass and sexual energy to make that particular plot point easy to overlook. Mixing the Cinderella theme with modern porn humor, the film gives us a prince seeking the perfect blow job, getting one at the ball, then sending his dedicated page boy out to be blown across the land until…well, you get the idea. Lighthearted fun is the theme here, the actors all clearly enjoy the sex, and the focus is on the women's pleasure as much as the men's.

DIRECTOR: Veronica Hart, 2002, 88 min.

CAST: Anita Cannibal, Bronze, Brooke Hunter, Julie Meadows, Michele Raven, Billy Glyde, Brick Majors, Cheyne Collins, Dale DaBone, Dillion Day, Ian Daniels, Joey Ray

Woman Penetrates Man

Natural Cast

Unsightly Boob Job

Well-Made Film

Real Female Orgasm

Still Insatiable

With tongue firmly in cheek, the legendary Marilyn Chambers returns after ten years to play a senator who campaigns on an antipornography platform. What she doesn't expect is that her crusade will turn her on, and her ethics take a back seat to her libido in a well-acted film with great dialogue and genuine sex.

DIRECTOR: Veronica Hart, 1999, 140 min.

CAST: Marilyn Chambers, Nikita, Jenteal, Vicca, Stacy Valentine, Kylie Ireland, Julia Ashton, Jullian, Tyce Bune, Jack Garfield, Steven St. Croix, Mr. Marcus

Sunset Stripped

Ginger Lynn stars in this excellent Veronica Hart–directed epic, an ode to Sunset Boulevard chock full of real female orgasms and hot hot sex. Ginger plays a writer, unable to create, sexually fixated on her agent, and totally out of money. When a repo man comes for her car, her life takes an unexpected turn as she winds up on the doorstep of an aged and insane male porn star from the "Golden Age." He puts her up in exchange for her editing skills on his autobiography, though she also has to participate in his weird nightly ritual that includes clothing from the 1980s—leotards best left forgotten. The sexy all-star cast (even the men!) puts in stunning performances all around, women call the shots in bed, the sex is genuinely intense, and the entire film is wonderfully watchable. The DVD contains interesting on-set interviews with the cast and Hart.

DIRECTOR: Veronica Hart, 2002, 137 min.

CAST: Alex Foxe, Ashlyn Gere, Chennin Blanc, Cheri, Ginger Lynn, Kelly Steele, Nikita Denis, Sharon Kane, Sondra Hall, Cheyne Collins, George Kaplan, Hamilton Steele, J. D. Coxxx, J. T. Cannon, Jamie Gillis, Mark Kernes, Mickey G, Randy Spears, Tyce Bune

The Swap 2
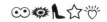

In a turnabout-is-fair-play, humorous look at monogamy and its frustrations, two attractive couples try swinging and the results, as in life, are unexpected. Well acted and engaging.

DIRECTOR: Paul Thomas, 1994, 72 min.

CAST: Dyanna Lauren, Asia Carrera, Leena, Isis Nile, Lene, Christina Angel, Veronica Sage, Chad Thomas, Marc Wallice, Alex Sanders, Brad Armstrong, Tony Tedeschi, Mark Davis

Dominant Women

Violet's Top Choice

Intense Chemistry

Extreme Sex Acts

Great for Newbies

Taken

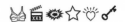

Ginger Lynn delivers a performance that goes far beyond many of her Hollywood counterparts in this controversial story about a woman who is abducted by a handsome stranger—and is sexually and emotionally seduced by him. Full, believable characters, suspense and drama, romance and passionate lovemaking, exciting sexual experimentation, and a surprise twist at the end are all part of this fantastic film.

DIRECTOR: Veronica Hart, 2001, 142 min.

CAST: Ginger Lynn, Herschel Savage, Evan Stone, Rebecca Lord, Alexandra Silk, Adajja, Tyler Wood, Kelsey, Randy Spears, Lexington Steele, George Kaplan

NOTE: Contains an internal ejaculation scene, won two *AVN* awards.

Taxi Dancers

A B-movie, but with a more complex plot than anything you'll see on TV, not to mention the raw sex. In an allusion to a time gone by, the film is set in an old-fashioned dance club, where dances are ten cents apiece. Our introduction to this seedy world is through the police investigation of a dancer's murder, which quickly uncovers underworld crime and results in a violent noir ending.

DIRECTOR: Paul Thomas, 1999, 111 min.

CAST: Angelica Sin, Asia Carrera, Jessica Darlin (nonsex), Leanni Lei (nonsex), Mickey, Rich Handsome, Tia Bella, Tim Hard, Tom Adams.

Thighs Wide Open

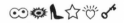

Chloe is married to a high-powered lawyer who is a two-timing jerk, and she's shut herself off sexually. They attend a party at his boss's house, where she is abandoned by her husband and chatted up by the boss, Randy Spears, whom (against her instincts) she follows upstairs and who subjects her to a scene from a porn film plus some intense verbal seduction. Later, he invites her back to attend a special party, and with the flirtation and tension cranked up, she shows up and they all but tear each other's clothes off on the stairs in a mesmerizing encounter. After that, she's led through a decadent sex party, and *we're* led through a lot of sex scenes—some hot, some not.

DIRECTOR: Fred J. Lincoln, 2001, 95 min.

CAST: Charlene Aspen, T. J. Hart, Bridgette Kerkove, Maya Divine, Justine Romee, Ronnie Coxx, Randy Spears, Kyle Stone, Evan Stone

Woman Penetrates Man

Natural Cast

Unsightly Boob Job

Well-Made Film

Real Female Orgasm

Tina Tyler's Going Down

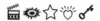

Written and directed by Tyler, this smart video cleverly crams wall-to-wall sex scenes into a neat little plot, making for a whole lotta sex in believable scenarios. Tyler herself plays a security guard who keeps an eye on the elevator through security cameras, though one car in particular seems to be the ideal spot for a number of heated trysts. When the passengers hit the "stop" button, Tyler watches and masturbates, and we get to see all the action. Favorite scenes include the opener with Nina Hartley and Sean Michaels, Tina's earth-shaking masturbation orgasm, and an interesting episode where a couple fights while two men quietly give each other hand jobs in the background. Excellent filming, editing, dialogue, and acting.

DIRECTOR: Tina Tyler, 2002, 74 min.

CAST: Nina Hartley, Kylie Ireland, Brooke Hunter, Kimi Lixx, Sean Michaels, Steve Hatcher, Tara Indiana, Dru Berrymore, Randy Spears

Unreal

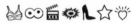

Chloe plays Monica English, a woman trapped in a life of manipulative men and her own quiet desperation. One morning she goes to the office and discovers the power to make sexual fantasies come true, finding her own personal power through her chaotic sexual machinations. As fantasy and reality blur, Monica's sanity becomes a subjective question, though it matters not when you watch the outstanding sex scenes on this tape. Great acting by all, and three sex scenes in particular—a yummy blow job, an outrageous girl–girl with Chloe and Tina Tyler, and a finale with Chloe and two anonymous men—make this film unforgettable. A little artsy at the end, but whatever.

DIRECTOR: Antonio Passolini, 2001, 112 min.

CAST: Chloe, Julie Meadows, Tina Tyler, Nicole Sheridan, Gina Ryder, Keri Windsor, Logan Labrent, Evan Stone, Mark Davis, Dillion Day, Randy Spears, Jean Luc Goddard, Voodoo

Dominant Women	Violet's Top Choice	Intense Chemistry	Extreme Sex Acts	Great for Newbies

Urban Friction
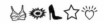

Set in Chicago, two modern lovers have agreed to make each other's number one sexual fantasy come true. In the prequel, *Thank You, Mistress,* punkette girlfriend Mika gave her boyfriend, Poochie, to a mistress, but this time it's Mika's turn and she's worried that her fantasy (being the cheese in a boy–boy sandwich) will break up her relationship. Meanwhile, her boyfriend has a fit of infidelity with a tattooed vixen, Mika masturbates, and she visits a very cute friend with very cute vibrators to relieve her tension. Great use of a low budget and terrific nonporn actors, with passionate sex and no formula—hooray!

DIRECTORS: Marianna Beck and Jack Hafferkamp, 2002, 75 min.

CAST: Mika, Poochie, others

NOTE: Independent filmmaker.

A Witch's Tail

Asia Carrera plays a frustrated writer who inherits an estate from her aunt, who, it turns out, was an evil witch who controlled the area for hundreds of years. Naïve Carrera is the unwitting sacrifice for her aunt's return and as the plot unfolds, several allies arrive to help—and have a lot of fun, energetic sex.

DIRECTOR: Bud Lee, 2000

CAST: Anna Malle, Asia Carrera, Alexandra Silk, Julie Meadows, Rayveness, Cheyenne Silver, Chris Cannon, Jon Dough, Joel Lawrence, Steve Hatcher

The Zone
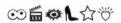

Explore a no-holds-barred sex club through the eyes of a frustrated divorcée, who gives us an eyeful. Searing scenes that include glory holes enjoyed by insatiable women, man-to-man sex, girl–girl sex with a transsexual woman, and more. Stylish and sophisticated, with sexually demanding women.

DIRECTOR: Paul Thomas, 1998, 90 min.

CAST: Dyanna Lauren, Stephanie Swift, Gina Rome, Kobe Tai, Ruby, Chloe Nicholle, Leah, Marcus Day, Devlin Weed, Mark Davis, Steven St. Croix, Paul Stryder, Michael Hurt, Julian St. Jox, Vince Voyeur, Mickey G, Tommy Gunn, Alex Sanders, Claudio, Jay Ashley

NOTE: Contains a lactation scene.

Woman Penetrates Man

Natural Cast

Unsightly Boob Job

Well-Made Film

Real Female Orgasm

The Classics: Porn's Golden Age

We wanted to see what all the fuss was about, so my boyfriend and I rented The Devil in Miss Jones. *Boy, were we surprised! The gory opening scene was something you'd never see in modern porn, and the sex went much further than we expected. It was a big turn-on for both of us.*

"Classic" or "Golden Age" porn encompasses adult videos made in the 1970s and 1980s. This term is also used when a particular film or video has a cultural or social significance, is notorious for one or more reasons, or has become a cult—or underground—favorite. Almost every film in this category was shot using film stock, for the camera technology, of course, predates the now-widespread use of digital cameras, and even VCRs. The real film stock gives these films a more movie-like feel and quality and, except for the nudity and explicit sex, makes them often indistinguishable from Hollywood films released at the same time.

It's not just the film stock that makes these films different, and a cut above the rest in movie-making terms, for porn made twenty-plus years ago was a whole different animal. Each feature was created to be projected onto a big screen in a movie theater, and more care was given to make a complete film. Plots were complex, actors were skilled and remarkable, and showing explicit sex was dealt with as an exciting taboo—one that performers were delighted to explore and enthusiastic to perform.

Explicit Time Capsules

By the late 1960s adult movies had settled comfortably into adult movie houses. These were old theaters that exclusively showed pornographic films, usually all day and evening long. The audience was primarily thought to be "raincoaters": men who slinked into the theaters to mas-turbate, though occasionally women and couples ventured in to do pretty much the same thing as the single guys. Porn was also watched at home on movie projectors or at "smokers" or "stag parties"—parties attended by single or married men, with no women. When *Deep Throat* was released, the attention it received sent mainstream America into the adult theaters in droves. Much of the attention came when bad-boy heartthrob Frank Sinatra used his own in-home movie projector in a private screening for Vice President Spiro Agnew.

An understanding of the culture at the time these films were made is crucial to appreciating the milieu of classic porn. In the early 1970s, the industry was on the cusp of an explosion, reveling in the fact that adult films were being made by people who saw their work as championing the free-speech provisions of the First Amendment to the Constitution. This attitude was fueled by the lifting of the archaic Motion Picture Production Code in 1968, resulting in greater freedom of expression for all filmmakers, and the subsequent release of Hollywood films depicting previously taboo themes (like *Rosemary's Baby*, 1968) and featuring a lot less clothing (such as *Barbarella*, also 1968). Porn actor Richard Pacheco soberingly adds that his generation at this time had a "take a pill mentality" about everything from syphilis to unwanted pregnancy. This was the beginning of the 1970s, and while Barbarella could bare her boobs and have orgasms in outer space, a conviction for being involved in a porn film could get you sent up for pimping and pandering, a three-year felony offense. Everyone who participated in adult films at this time stuck together. They'd meet at restaurants and move to undisclosed locations for shooting.

Beauty standards as seen in popular culture were different then. Makeup, hair, and clothes were worn differently, shaving and waxing body hair were not yet trends, and surgical augmentation was rare. The subject matter sometimes followed along taboo lines that today's filmmakers—both adult and nonerotic—wouldn't dare explore. Staying true to plot and character, directors depicted explicit violence right alongside the sex, something you'd never see in today's cautious adult features. Incest, rape, and loss of virginity were not-uncommon themes, and entire features such as the famous *Behind the Green Door* were about women who were kidnapped and forced into sexual servitude. These films were far from politically correct—racial stereotypes were prevalent and female characters were often coerced into nonconsensual sexual situations.

All the same, you can find classic porn with no taboo themes whatsoever, such as elaborate musicals, with song, dance, great costumes—*and* hot sex. Or thoughtful, intense explorations of relationships, with emotions running the gamut of human expression. Films could be goofy, fun, and light, but could turn dirty and explicit as viewers followed the exploits of giggling cheerleaders, desperately horny candy stripers, or sexually demanding housewives. Also, the lines between porn and Hollywood cinema became blurred for a short period, producing films such as *Caligula,* as well as cult crossover hits like *Café Flesh.*

Classic Porn Directors

Just as with any film, each classic adult film bears the individual stamp of the director. Direction style, cinematography, editing, the way script and plot were communicated to the viewer, and the performance of the actors all depended on the vision and synthesis of the director's overall concept for the film. In classic porn—where these things were prized highly—this was especially true. Also, because feature-length porn was in its fledgling stage, directors from porn's Golden Age often came from film back-grounds or worked in the film industry, whereas now porn directors often learn film from within porn but have little outside film experience. Classic porn directors not only possessed well-rounded film experience, such as Robert McCallum (who worked as Orson Welles's cameraman for fif-teen years), but also cited a variety of artistic influences on their work, such as Radley Metzger (aka Henry Paris), who was heavily influenced by art-house directors like Buñuel and Bergman.

Joe D'Amato

Italian cult director Joe D'Amato was one of the kings of "splatter films," a true master of the graphic blood-, violence-, and sex-drenched Italian B-movie, though he also made porn films that were some of the most highly regarded adult films of all time. He was the cult director's expert everyman, and worked in every genre of film imaginable, including west-ern, vampire, convent/horny nun, women in prison, sword and sandal, cannibals, postapocalypse, and more. He loved to imitate popular culture with his films, and would create low-budget, though outrageously over-the-top, productions of everything he could. In Europe, cult directors like D'Amato were viewed differently than their counterparts in America , and though many of D'Amato's films were low-budget cult flicks, throughout the course of his prolific career he worked with such illustrious names as Sam Neill, Klaus Kinski, master composer Ennio Morricone, and cine-matographer Aristide Massacce. He was affectionately known (okay, maybe not by everyone) as "Italy's worst director," though when he began making porn, his films exceeded the standards and even received great reviews, largely for the fantastic cinematography and excellent framing. Just before his fatal heart attack in 1999, he stated that he wanted to leave porn and return to his extreme-gore days, circa 1980. His adult features won several *AVN* awards.

Robert McCallum

This prolific filmmaker made some of the best classic porn in history, bringing to the genre both a professional eye and a knack for capturing the perfect, subtle shot. He was known in nonerotic cinema by his real name, Gary Graver, and worked as a cinematographer on several cult exploitation films such as *I Spit on Your Corpse* and *Invasion of the Bee Girls*. He was a filmmaker since the early 1960s, when he graduated from Los Angeles City College, and though he studied acting with Bruce Dern, Jeff Corey, and Lee J. Cobb, he felt his calling was on the other side of the camera, as a director. Exploitation and sexploitation films became his standard, till in the early 1970s he caught the attention of Orson Welles, who used Graver for fifteen years, making him director of photography on all of Welles's film and TV projects. His first porn film was *Three a.m.* (1975), and one of his adult film career highlights was *Amanda by Night*. While all this was happening, he continued to make films under the McCallum moniker, even into the early 1990s when he became a high-demand second unit director on films such as *Enter the Dragon* and *Raiders of the Lost Ark*. Graver's films from the late 1970s and early 1980s are his best adult work, and it's remarkable to think that there is one person who can say that they've worked with both Marilyn Chambers and Orson Welles.

Henry Paris, aka Radley Metzger

Creating adult masterpieces under two names, this director created the most distinctive and artful adult feature films ever made. His work was very European in character, and was in fact often shot in Europe, though it usually featured highly skilled American actors who were not afraid to go all the way when it came to sex. These were regular films, after all, but with sex in them. As Radley Metzger he made films that crossed over into nonerotic cinema, pushing the boundaries of sex in film, and shot films that were elegant, erotic, provocative, and shocking by the standards of the 1960s and early 1970s. He was a native New Yorker whose love for film purportedly came from the hours he spent in movie theaters to find relief from his allergies thanks to their air conditioning. He started out doing commercials and cutting films for Janus Films, which exposed him to filmmakers such as Ingmar Bergman, François Truffaut, and others. He began making his unique dramatic/erotic films in 1957, with *Dark Odyssey*, and went on to create soft-core works of art with *The Dirty Girls, The Alley Cats, Therese and Isabelle, Camille 2000, The Lickerish Quartet,* and *Score* (the latter released in both soft- and hard-core versions). He made only five hard-core films, but they were some of the best adult films ever made. He now studies homeopathic medicine.

Classic Porn Reviews

The list of classic films available is lengthy, and if you like their cinematic quality and the fresh enthusiasm of the sex play, you'll have a lot to explore. This chapter gets you started, covering the highest-quality classics and including all the well-known epics.

3 a.m.

Professional cinematography and great casting frame this terrific exploration of intergenerational relationships—and their conflicts—through the eyes of a young woman. Georgina Spelvin plays a woman having an affair with her brother-in-law, causing an uproar in the whole family. The original alluded to an incest relationship, but any copy you find will have these references edited out.

DIRECTOR: Robert McCallum, 1975, 90 min.

CAST: Georgina Spelvin, Rhonda Gellard, Sharon Thorpe, Clara Dia, Rob Rose, Judith Hamilton, Charles Hooper

7 Into Snowy

The title lets you know that this is a modern (at the time) spin on the *Snow White* theme, but with a decidedly adult twist. Busty Kay Parker is innocent Snowy, whose evil stepmother hates her because the magic mirror doesn't lie. The stepmother seduces men to abuse Snowy and leave her for dead, but Snowy's abundant charms save the day, and the guys fall for Snowy.

DIRECTOR: Antonio Sheppard, 1977, 80 min.

CAST: Abigail Clayton, Kay Parker, Paul Thomas, John Leslie, Turk Lyon

Woman Penetrates Man

Natural Cast

Unsightly Boob Job

Well-Made Film

Real Female Orgasm

Alice in Wonderland

You have to see this one to believe that a porn musical is even possible—and could turn out perfect and hilarious. Elaborate costuming, great filming, and skilled actors sing, dance, and screw their way through Carroll's classic tale. What's more, the sex is sincere and full of chemistry. It's a weird, wonderful world we live in, and this is the proof. And yes, Tweedledee and Tweedledum are real-life husband and wife. Beware of the softer "R" version and look for the longer X-rated tape.

DIRECTOR: Bud Townsend, 1976, 81 min.

CAST: Kristine DeBell, Bradford Armdexter, Gila Havana, Ron Nelson, Alan Novak, J. P. Paradine, Jerry Spelman, Sue Tsengoles, Tony Tsengoles, Angel Barrett, Nancy Dare, Bruce Finklesteen, Juliet Graham, Terri Hall, Astrid Hayase

NOTE: Cult classic.

Amanda by Night; Amanda by Night 2

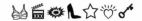

Veronica Hart is a high-class prostitute trying to start a new life when an old friend asks for a final favor, so she sets up a scene and winds up in the middle of a murder. A complete film with a real plot, and actors that make it work. Has a great domination scene and a very dangerous Jamie Gillis as an eerie turn-on, not to mention that Veronica Hart is mesmerizing. In #2, Hart returns as a reformed prostitute who runs a counseling service for sex workers. She finds herself again at the nexus of a murder investigation, this time as a liaison to help the cop find his call girl, who is caught in the middle of an organized crime web. A sex-fueled mystery worthy of its excellent predecessor.

Amanda by Night

DIRECTOR: Robert McCallum, 1982, 95 min.

CAST: Veronica Hart, Lisa De Leeuw, Jamie Gillis, Ron Jeremy, others

Amanda by Night 2

DIRECTOR: Jack Remy, 1988, 85 min.

CAST: Krista Lane, Nina Hartley, Veronica Hart, Tracey Adams, Nikki Knights

NOTE: Won an *AVN* award.

| Dominant Women | Violet's Top Choice | Intense Chemistry | Extreme Sex Acts | Great for Newbies |

Autobiography of a Flea

With faultless period costuming and lots of sacrilegious references, this liberal adaptation of the smutty classic told from the point of view of a pubic hair flea is a presentation of Victorian debauchery at its finest. Good acting, bad acting, taboo themes, and a bunch of very horny (and very famous) actors make it worthwhile. As with many classic adult films it handles a theme that directors today would debate until blue in the face—the plot centers on a young girl who is so alluring that all the men try to rape her, and she instead flips them and screws them with insatiable lust. Quite a fantasy, but *whose* fantasy is up for grabs.

DIRECTOR: Sharon MacNight, 1984, 93 min.

CAST: Annette Haven, Jean Jennings, John Leslie, Paul Thomas, John Holmes

NOTE: A Mitchell Brothers production.

Bad Penny

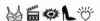

Sexy Samantha Fox stars as a woman who must solve the hokey riddle her father left behind in his will in order to inherit his fortune: "What is French, turns on at night, and gives good crown?" Thing is, she's a bimbo and must beat her evil aunt to the punch, and when she finds out her uncle in New York can help, she winds up doing research for the answer in a fancy Manhattan sex club. Terrific production values and a great sex-club scene.

DIRECTOR: Chuck Vincent, 1978, 80 min.

CAST: Samantha Fox, Robert Bolla, Kurt Mann, Dave Ruby, Don Peterson, Roger Caine, Georgette Sanders, Adam DeHaven, Clea Carson, Paula Morton, Robin Byrd, Anna St. James, Allstyne Von Busch, Karl Murdoch, Ben Pierce, Tony Mansfield, Peter Ross, Maxwell Maximum, Charlie Briggs, Adam DeHaven, Hector Morales, David Morris

| Woman Penetrates Man | Natural Cast | Unsightly Boob Job | Well-Made Film | Real Female Orgasm |

Barbara Broadcast

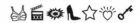

One of the most beautiful adult actresses of all time, Annette Haven, plays Barbara Broadcast, a celebrity call girl and a best-selling sex author who is the subject of a reporter's story and affections. The far-above-average production values showcase the surreal but incredibly sexy and whimsical atmosphere, whether Haven is dining sweetly at a sex-filled restaurant (on appetizers and tastes of waiters) or having a frenzied girl–girl in a disco. Tenderness and a bit of kink, plus an unsurpassed cinematic style, make this an outstanding film.

DIRECTOR: Henry Paris, 1977, 90 min.

CAST: Annette Haven, C. J. Laing, Constance Money, Suzanne McBaine, Jamie Gillis

NOTE: Cult classic.

Behind the Green Door

Although it's one of the most famous films of all time, many people forget that it's a tale of abduction and forced sexual performances, containing many themes that still shock today and turned audiences' hair white at its 1973 release. America had to go straight to a shrink and get on the couch after pure, snow-white Marilyn Chambers is kidnapped and "loses" her virginity to a huge, outrageously stereotypical black stud on a stage, and she is subjected to pretty much every sexual scenario that could press a button. Little dialogue and many much-talked-about scenes. The film took its namesake from the famous "Green Door" massage parlor in San Francisco's North Beach, which still stands today.

DIRECTOR: Artie and Jim Mitchell, 1973, 68 min.

CAST: Adrienne Mitchell (nonsex), Angela Castle, Ariel Porny, Bunnie Brody, Barbara Bryan, Bernice Mago, Bonnie Parker, Marilyn Chambers, Hadley von Baxendale, Jan Hartman, Kandi Johnson, Linda Chapman, Linda Grant, Letitia Torrez, Martha Strawberry, Mira Vane, Nancy Wilson, Rabin Drantha, Artie Mitchell (nonsex), Ben Davidson, Bill Hadley, Barry Vane, Dale Meador, George Marconi, George S. McDonald, Jerry Ross, Johnnie Keyes, Jim Mitchell (nonsex), Kurt Hartman, M Bradford, Michael Gebe, Mick Jones, Richard Coburn, Rick Dayton, Tom Cloud, Ted McKnight, Tony Royalle, Tyler Reynolds, Yank Levine

NOTE: Cult classic.

Dominant Women   Violet's Top Choice   Intense Chemistry   Extreme Sex Acts   Great for Newbies

Café Flesh

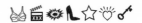

This artsy, futuristic adult film was a cult classic at a time when sci-fi and movies about the future were a big staple in mainstream entertainment. In the aftermath of World War III, the "nuclear kiss" has left 99 percent of the population "sex negatives," unable to derive pleasure from sex, or even to *have* it. The tiny 1 percent who can have pleasurable sex are required by the government to perform sex onstage for the wealthy, elite "negatives." A negative couple is fixated by the shows at Café Flesh, but when they try it at home, they become violently ill. Except that Lana, the woman in the couple, is faking it—and here's where our story begins. The *Cabaret*-style atmosphere holds our attention throughout the film, and the somewhat short-lived sex acts are outstanding.

DIRECTOR: Rinse Dream, 1983, 90 min.

CAST: Pia Snow, Marie Sharp, Kevin James, Andrew Nichols

NOTE: Screenplay by Jerry Stahl, who wrote *Permanent Midnight,* won an AVN award in 1983. Cult classic.

Caligula

This was allegedly the most lavish, costly, and elaborate production to ever feature hard-core sex, and it is an important film in many ways, most especially because it features such major stars—Peter O'Toole, Sir John Gielgud, and Helen Mirren. It is not, however, for the faint of heart as it contains a lot of graphic violence, much of it sexual. Unlike standard erotic film, it does not contain wall-to-wall sex, whether in close-up or for extended scenes, but instead edits the sex tastefully and distributes it in small, script-appropriate doses. Bob Guccione (*Penthouse* magazine) helmed the production, and because he wanted to give the film more punch, much of the hard sex scenes were shot and edited in after the fact—unbeknownst to the major actors. The film chronicles the historical figure of Emperor Caligula of Rome, whose spiral into madness was legendary because of the atrocities he personally perpetrated on those around him. Most notable in the sex realm is the unprompted, unscripted lesbian scene between two *Penthouse* pets who were actually lovers at the time.

DIRECTOR: Tinto Brass, 1979, 148 min.

CAST: Helen Mirren, Teresa Ann Savoy, Anneka Di Lorenzo, Lori Wagner, Adriana Asti, Leopoldo Trieste, Giancarlo Badessi, Mirella Dangelo, John Gielgud, Malcolm McDowell, Paolo Bonacelli, Guido Mannari, John Steiner, Peter O'Toole

NOTE: Cult classic.

Woman Penetrates Man

Natural Cast

Unsightly Boob Job

Well-Made Film

Real Female Orgasm

THE CLASSICS: PORN'S GOLDEN AGE • 149

Candy Stripers

Goofy and fun, and full of enthusiastic sex, *Candy Stripers* sets the scene when three young horny women decide to spread their own brand of good cheer throughout a hospital. Naughty nurses, lucky patients, doctors perfecting their "stroke," and more are all in this terrific, stimulating little film. Light fare, with lots of smiling performers.

DIRECTOR: Bob Chinn, 1978, 82 min.

CAST: Mimi Morgan, Eileen Wells, Cris Cassidy, Nancy Hoffman, Amber Hunt, Lauren Black, Sharon Thorpe, Pheadra Grant, Bron White, Paul Thomas, Richard Pacheco, Joey Silvera, Don Fernando, Rock Steadie, David Clark

NOTE: The original version contained a fisting scene that has been edited out, has one giant orgy, and has an all-girl group sex scene at the end.

Cinderella

Another…musical? You bet! But this one, though difficult to find, stands head and shoulders above *Alice in Wonderland,* in every respect, delivering steamy sex, great musical numbers, and hilarious porno-fied caricatures of the Cinderella characters. Cinderella is on the usual quest to escape cruel stepsisters and catch the prince, except that her fairy godmother is a bitchy diva queen—a black transvestite—who gives Cinderella a unique qualification to catch the prince's attention: a snapping pussy. Yes, you read that right: Her pussy snaps in rhythm when she's turned on, and the prince must find the pussy that fits his penis and snaps in time to know which of the women was his dream girl. Full of painfully bad one-liners; great for an intentionally hilarious night of unintentionally bad cinema.

DIRECTOR: Michael Pataki, 1977, 78 min.

CAST: Cheryl Smith, Sy Richardson, Brett Smiley, others

NOTE: Cult classic.

Dominant Women

Violet's Top Choice

Intense Chemistry

Extreme Sex Acts

Great for Newbies

Debbie Does Dallas

Gals of today going for the retro look should take notes while watching this film, which is fun, kitschy, and campy while displaying all the styles we love to hate about the 1970s—feathered blonde hair, cords and polyester, and oh, the music, yikes. Debbie is a star cheerleader who's earned a spot on a professional team, but can't afford to get to Dallas—until her bubbly cheerleading pals put together "Teen Services," a business that provides clients with oral satisfaction. Plenty of cheerleaders, football players, and locker room sex adventures.

DIRECTOR: Jim Clark, 1978, 83 min.

CAST: Arcadia Lake, Bambi Woods, Christie Ford, Debbie Lewis, Georgette Saunders, Jenny Cole, Kasey Rodgers (nonsex), Merle Michaels, Robin Byrd, Rikki O'Neal, Ben Pierce (nonsex), David Morris, David Sutton, Eric Edwards, Hershel Savage, Jack Teague (nonsex), Peter Lerman, R. Bolla, Steve Marshall, Tony Mansfield

Deep Throat

This was the film that brought porn into the collective consciousness and drew thousands of people to XXX theaters who had never previously seen a porn film—and over the years became the center for hot debate about women's roles as performers in porn. Linda Lovelace plays a woman who can't get off until her pervy doctor discovers that her clitoris is actually in her throat, paving the way for Linda to showcase her amazing sword-swallowing abilities through-out the film. Lots and lots and *lots* of blow jobs.

DIRECTOR: Gerard Damiano, 1972, 62 min.

CAST: Carol Connors, Dolly Sharp, Linda Lovelace, Bill Harrison, Bob Phillips, Gerald Damiano (nonsex), Harry Reems, John Byron, Michael Powers, Ted Street, William Love

NOTE: Folks afraid of 1970s pubic hair will be elated to know that Lovelace is shaved in this film. Cult classic.

| Woman Penetrates Man | Natural Cast | Unsightly Boob Job | Well-Made Film | Real Female Orgasm |

Devil in Miss Jones

Another well-known film with macabre and potentially disturbing themes: the opening scene finds a woman—Justine Jones, a virgin spinster—in a bathtub committing a gruesome, bloody suicide. She goes to Purgatory where she makes a deal with the devil for more time, as long as she's "consumed by lust." No problem for Georgina Spelvin, whose tangible pleasure in every sex act she participates in is refreshing. Not as many genital close-ups as other films, and the background music is mellow and unobtrusive.

DIRECTOR: Gerard Damiano, 1972, 62 min.

CAST: Erica Havens, Judith Hamilton, Georgina Spelvin, Gerald Damiano (non-sex), Harry Reems, John Clemens (nonsex), Levi Richards, Marc Stevens

NOTE: Has a DP with Spelvin. Cult classic.

Dracula Exotica

Hammer Horror could never go this far, but *Dracula Exotica* plays 1970s-style Dracula to the hilt (even though it's a 1980 release). With wit, humor, a flair for drama, and a good amount of fetish thrown in for excitement, this version of *Dracula* finds the count fleeing to America to evade Hungarian tax collectors—there, he's suspected of being a spy and a murderer. The acting and sex are superb, and I found myself looking forward to the next sex scene, rather than preparing myself for the predictable. This film showcases Vanessa del Rio in one of her best roles.

DIRECTOR: Warren Evans, 1980, 98 min.

CAST: Christine deShaffer, Vanessa del Rio, Denise Sloan, Diane Sloan, Samantha Fox, Terry Yale (nonsex), Marlene Willoughby, Bobby Astyr, David Ruby, Eric Edwards, Gordon Duvall (nonsex), Hershel Savage, Jamie Gillis, Roger Caine, Ron Hudd, Ron Jeremy, Randy West

Dominant Women

Violet's Top Choice

Intense Chemistry

Extreme Sex Acts

Great for Newbies

Emmanuelle

This soft-core Columbia Pictures classic, based on the notorious novel, rarely makes it onto any politically correct, recommended viewing lists owing to its theme and its sometimes disturbing depiction of sex acts, though it stays true to the original story and premise. Emmanuelle is married to the ambassador of Thailand, and when she expresses her boredom, he suggests that she take advantage of their open relationship. She does just that, and embarks on a series of sexual experiences that finish with her in the position of existing solely to give pleasure to others, at the whims of the male characters. For those who enjoy well-built films and female sexual submissives, this film's a prize, though there is a soft rape scene in the context of her "education" and other nonconsensual displays with Emmanuelle as the object. Perhaps this film is best known for the scene where a woman in a bar smokes a cigarette with her vagina. Shot on location in Thailand.

DIRECTOR: Just Jaeckin, 1973, 94 min.

CAST: Sylvia Kristel, Marika Green, Jeanne Colletin, Christine Boisson, Daniel Sarky, Alain Cuny

NOTE: Foreign release. Cult classic.

The Grafenberg Spot

Lighthearted and by no means an educational treatise on the G-spot or female ejaculation, this film focuses on female orgasm as it pretends to explore the phenomenon of the G-spot. Male come shots are rare in it, and female ejaculation is the name of the game, though several of the "squirting" shots are inauthentic (but many of the female orgasms are). Hilarious and fun, with an all-star cast at its sex-lovin' best. Best of luck finding a version with the underage Traci Lords scene still intact.

DIRECTOR: Jim and Artie Mitchell, 1985, 75 min.

CAST: Harry Reems, Ginger Lynn, Annette Haven, Fanny Fatale, Amber Lynn, Nina Hartley, John Holmes, Lili Marlene, Rick Savage, Rita Ricardo, Traci Lords, Thor Southern

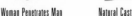
Woman Penetrates Man

Natural Cast

Unsightly Boob Job

Well-Made Film

Real Female Orgasm

History of the Blue Movie

With silent stag loops of the 1910s and '20s, explicit cartoons from the '30s, shorts of the '40s and '50s, and explicit material from the '60s and '70s, this collection of erotic film samples is more entertaining and enlightening to watch than it is erotic, though many of the scenes are rather exciting. No music or dialogue, so you're left to your own conclusions, but at least you can give it any sound track you like.

DIRECTOR: Alex DeRenzy, 1983, 108 min.

CAST: N/A

Insatiable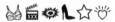

Marilyn Chambers plays a woman who has inherited a fortune after her parents' deaths, but realizes that money can't fill the void she's feeling and decides that what she needs is a good lay. Except she can't find the perfect partner, which sets the stage for the beautiful and sexually rapacious Chambers to demonstrate why she was a star unparalleled by today's new talent. Like many films of its day it has an archetypal scene where virgin teen Chambers loses her virginity to the gardener, but unlike the others it's a juicy, panties-around-the ankles showstopper.

DIRECTOR: Robert McCallum, 1980, 80 min.

CAST: Marilyn Chambers, John Holmes, Mike Ranger, Serena, David Morris, Jessie St. James, Richard Pacheco, John Leslie, Joan Turner.

NOTE: Cult classic.

Naked Came the Stranger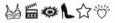

Gillian and William are a monogamous heterosexual couple who run a morning radio talk show, but when Gillian finds her husband in *flagrante* and gushing repugnant baby talk to the production assistant, she's furious—and turned on. What ensues is her personal sexual explorations to boost her ego in the light of her husband's infidelity, creating an unrushed, complex drama.

DIRECTOR: Henry Paris, 1985, 75 min.

CAST: Darbi Rains, Mary Stuart, Levi Richards

Dominant Women

Violet's Top Choice

Intense Chemistry

Extreme Sex Acts

Great for Newbies

New Wave Hookers

Lowbrow production values, enormous 1980s hair, garish outfits, and an outrageously lame premise make this a classic for perhaps some very unintentional reasons. Two guys decide to become pimps: That's it. The rest is yellow suits, roller-skating hookers, new wave music (some by The Plugz, who were later on the *Repo Man* sound track), and uninspired sex. The original contained an underage Traci Lords, though you'd better believe her scene has been edited out.

DIRECTOR: Gregory Dark, 1985, 60 min.

CAST: Ginger Lynn, Gina Carrera, Desiree Lane, Kristara Barrington, Kimberly Carson, Brooke Fields, Jamie Gillis, Traci Lords, Jake Baker

NOTE: Cult classic.

Only the Best 1 and 2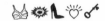

If all you want is a collection of critics' choice scenes from classic 1970s and 1980s porn, then these tapes compiled by adult film historian Jim Holliday are just what the doctor ordered. A terrific selection containing a variety of sex acts, authentic female orgasms, and fantastic chemistry between partners.

DIRECTOR, VOL. 1: Jim Holliday, 1986, 105 min.

DIRECTOR, VOL. 2: Jim Holliday, 1989, 80 min.

Opening of Misty Beethoven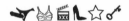

Jamie Gillis is a writer who, as research for a book he's working on, seeks out the most uninspired prostitute he can find and aims to make her the most respected and sought-after call girl in Europe. Gillis's rich friends will spare no expense in her training, creating the most outrageous and extravagant scenarios for her erotic "tests." It's a lavishly told version of *My Fair Lady* that has all the hallmarks of terrific classic porn: believable acting, great cinematography, a fun story, and performers who really get into the sex.

DIRECTOR: Henry Paris, 1976, 86 min.

CAST: Constance Money, Jacqueline Beudant, Gloria Leonard, Terry Hall, Jamie Gillis

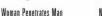

Woman Penetrates Man   Natural Cast   Unsightly Boob Job   Well-Made Film   Real Female Orgasm

Other Side of Julie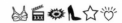

A great John Leslie vehicle with all the early 1980s-era trappings, though with a slightly more sophisticated feel than its classic porn counterparts. The sex is heated and the scenes are sensuous and unhurried, with the overall production filmed with thoughtful pacing and care that just isn't found in most adult film. John Leslie's wife is sexually frustrated, mostly because he's out having affairs all over the place, so she experiments on her own to find satisfaction.

DIRECTOR: Anthony Riverton, 1981, 83 min.

CAST: Nancy Hoffman, Susannah French, Kristine Heller, Gloria Roberts, John Leslie

Outlaw Ladies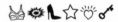

These housewives aren't bored—they've got their own daytime sex club to keep them busy! This film earns high ratings not for lavish sets or high budgets, but for the tasteful and arousing way in which the women's quest for sexual satisfaction is handled. It's all about women who know what they want, and use the men as living sex toys to get off. No complex plot, just lots of sincere, sizzling sex.

DIRECTOR: Henri Pachard, 1981, 83 min.

CAST: Veronica Hart, Juliet Anderson, Samantha Foxx, Marlene Willoghby, Merle Michaels, Jody Maxwell, Bobby Astyr, Richard Bolla, John Leslie

Private Afternoons of Pamela Mann

With his trademark beautiful camera work, quirky and ironic—yet utterly authentic—characters, and high production values, director Paris creates an atmosphere of absurdity and sexual rapture unseen in porn today. A husband is obsessed with what his wife is up to during the day, so he hires a private detective to follow her around. The detective gets an eyeful of her nonstop sexual activities, including many mouth-watering blow jobs and plenty of female orgasms—though Pamela herself never gets off.

DIRECTOR: Henry Paris, 1974, 83 min.

CAST: Barbara Bourbon, Darby Lloyd Rains, Kevin Andre, Eric Edwards, Sonny Landham

Dominant Women　　Violet's Top Choice　　Intense Chemistry　　Extreme Sex Acts　　Great for Newbies

Score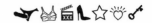

A pair of dope-smokin' swingers are vacationing in the French Riviera (actually Yugoslavia) at a rented house, where they play out their kinky sexual fantasies around wagers of who can seduce straight folks into taking a walk on the wild side. Fun, hilarious, and populated with the best unheard-of actors in soft core, this film is a favorite because of the humorous handling of all the archetypes and excellent storytelling. Also wonderful because it contains every type of pairing you'd imagine, is mature and ironic, and pits self-imposed chaste ideals against human curiosity and desire.

DIRECTOR: Radley Metzger, 1972, 86 min.

CAST: Claire Wilbur, Gerald Grant, Cal Culver (aka the late gay porn star Casey Donovan), Lynn Lowry

NOTE: Light S/M activities with sex.

Sex World

This fun spoof of *Westworld* charts the course of a busload of people en route to a resort that promises to help rid them of their sexual hang-ups. They're all carefully monitored and charted by lab-coated technicians who pair the lovers in situations that challenge their repressed desires, and show a hilarious and sexy tension between lovers whose worlds are purposely colliding, including lovers of different colors.

DIRECTOR: Anthony Thornberg, 1985, 90 min.

CAST: Leslie Bovee, Annette Haven, Sharon Thorpe, Kay Parker, Desiree West, John Leslie, Kent Hall, Jack Wright, Amber Hunt, Abigail Clayton, Cris Cassidy, Joey Silvera, Johnnie Keyes, Carol Tong, Roberto Ramos, Peter Johns, Maureen Spring

| Woman Penetrates Man | Natural Cast | Unsightly Boob Job | Well-Made Film | Real Female Orgasm |

The Story of O

Following along the story line of Pauline Réage's famous, banned, and best-selling erotic manuscript, the film follows a young woman, called only "O," who will do anything to prove her loyalty and submission to her master, so that she may belong to him entirely. While it's barely soft core, it goes all the way when showing erotic BDSM, including plenty of whips, chains, restraints, and worshipful sexual favors, though without any graphic sexual close-ups.

DIRECTOR: Just Jaekin, 1984, 96 min.

CAST: Corinne Clery, Christine Minazsoli, Anthony Steel, Alain Noruy

NOTE: Cult classic. S/M activities with sex.

Sweet Alice

When his wife disappears, a young studly cowboy hires a sexy but no-nonsense private detective to find her, and their search leads them all the way to Los Angeles. The pair wind up trolling the adult film industry to find the wife, taking the viewer on a virtual tour of porn sets and stars of the day, concluding when they find her in the center of a huge orgy. No expense was spared, and the casting is terrific.

DIRECTOR: Adele Robbins, 1983, 75 min.

CAST: Seka, John Holmes, Desirée Cousteau, Jamie Gillis, Kevin James, Honey Wilder, Paul Thomas, Becky Savage, Mike Eyke, Drea, Bill Margold

V: The Hot One
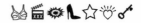

A splendid cast, great cinematography, and loads of hot, raunchy sex make this complex drama one of the best classics available today. Annette Haven is married to high-powered lawyer John Leslie, and together the couple appear cool and sophisticated. But on the inside, Haven is on fire with lust for any quick, dirty, and nasty sexual escapade she can get herself into.

DIRECTOR: Robert McCallum, 1984, 89 min.

CAST: Annette Haven, Laurien Dominique, Desiree West, Kay Parker, Paul Thomas, John Leslie, Joey Silvera

 Dominant Women   Violet's Top Choice   Intense Chemistry   Extreme Sex Acts   Great for Newbies

8

All Sex, No Plot

All I have to do is watch a blow job or a facial come shot—I don't need a story. I don't even need a dildo or vibrator.

All-sex films capture hot, one-time-only sex while it's really happening, with unscripted performances that show you what actually took place. The sex can be deliciously concentrated: thigh-shaking, white-knuckle rides through real female orgasms, chemistry that will have you picking your jaw up off the floor—and you're right there for every tasty minute. No bad acting, no plot to distract you. All-sex films are exactly that: all sex, with no distractions like acting, believability, sets, or frills. Most all-sex videos, especially the gonzo variety, are the "reality TV" of porn.

Videos with no plot and wall-to-wall sex are the ultimate instant-gratification visual sex toy. People who don't care about story line or characterization can cut right to the chase when they pick up one of these tapes and get exactly what they're looking for—graphic sex, and nothing else. These tapes sandwich one tasty sex scene after another, making them suitable for repeat use, like a favorite sex toy. The viewer can play one scene, stop the tape, and come back to try out the next scene later without feeling compelled to finish the story—and each new scene can be like a treat that you enjoy privately, just for yourself or with your honey. And if you find a favorite scene that bears repeat masturbation use, like a favorite fantasy, you won't have to guess about its location in the plot on the tape or DVD chapter. You can just replay your fantasy until you're spent.

All-sex films often suggest a theme that knits together a tape or a series, and the individual scenes may be strung over a scenario or have a hint of fantasy elements to rev your engine. Such themes can be a viewer fantasy, such as voyeurism, in which case the cameraman sets up the scene as if watching through a window, from behind bushes, or from the perspective of a taxicab driver watching his fare in the rearview mirror. A theme can be the first-time performance of an actor, having sex with other performers, the cameraman, or solo. Or it can be the sex act itself: oral sex, multiple male partners, couples. All-sex videos can focus on a particular female performer, such as the *Deep Inside* series, where the actress introduces her favorite scenes. Or they can be compilations of scenes from other tapes. If you are turned on by one particular type of sex, you can find a film that features it exclusively.

"Gonzo" porn is all sex, but filmed in a *cinema verité* style. By the end of the 1980s, porn makers didn't need a big budget to make porn—just a camera. It seemed no longer necessary, and not at all practical, to create high-quality adult films like those that had screened in theaters. Demand for porn continued to increase, yet with the increasing ease of production the quality of porn paradoxically plummeted. Practically anyone could churn out several films a week—and still can. In 1989 a new genre was born: "gonzo," where no plot is required and the person with the camera directs the action, occasionally getting involved and giving the viewer a first-person experience. Taking its name from Hunter S. Thompson's irreverent, improvised situational style of journalism, the genre gave every camcorder owner the feeling he or she could make porn, and elevated voyeurism into a style of video production. John Stagliano (aka "Buttman") and Ed Powers pioneered gonzo and are considered by many to be at the top of the trade, though they now share the field with talented film-makers such as Adam Glasser (Seymore Butts) and Ben Dover.

While past technological breakthroughs like VCRs and camcorders—and new ones like streaming video over the Web, inexpensive digital video, and satellite/cable accessibility—have lowered the level of cine-matic quality in porn, they've also turned up the sexual heat. Gonzo done well can capture plenty of unscripted, incredible sex scenes. Gonzo often uses amateurs, whose enthusiasm and freshness can be arresting. Wall-to-wall, all-sex porn occasionally overlaps into gonzo, and the result is videos where the cameraman directs and talks only occasionally. Either way, these videos can be highly arousing. The *Screaming Orgasms* series is a great example, and my top pick for couples-themed all-sex videos is the *Amateur Angels* series. The whole style of plotless voyeur porn can make for absolutely the best masturbation material, for many of the same reasons. You can see the arousing results in John Leslie's exceptional *Voyeur* and *Fresh Meat* videos.

Still, it's tougher today than it was thirty years ago to find a full-length feature that stands up to high-quality stroke classics like *Outlaw Ladies* and *The Opening of Misty Beethoven*. But even though a whole lot of bad new porn is now flooding the market, plenty of gems continue to be produced as a result of the industry's change and growth. In fact, because of tech-nology's impact on how much the viewer controls what she or he sees, adult filmmakers and distributors alike are starting to truly hone the films to meet the market's demand for good videos, intense sex, believability, and actors-as-real-people who reflect who we are and what we lust after.

All-Sex Directors

Although all-sex films seem to follow a simple formula—a man or woman with a camera shoots people having sex—the all-sex films available range widely in type and quality, according to who is behind the camera. All-sex films can be glossy, polished, and sleek, like those made by Andrew Blake, or rough and gritty, like films by Joe Gallant. There seem to be more all-sex directors than fish in the sea, and what follows is by no means a complete list—just a list of the best. So, to see all-sex action, filmed the way you'd like to see it, read on.

Andrew Blake (wall-to-wall)

Ever want to see a *Playboy* centerfold come to life? That's exactly what an Andrew Blake film is like but way, way better. The women are drop-dead gorgeous in every detail and, in my experience, unlike many other starlets, just as beautiful in real life. It's like watching supermodels with well-proportioned bodies preen, pout, wear sexy fetish outfits and lingerie... and then jump into sex in scenes and sets that are visually stunning. Whenever a male is present, he's pretty much used as a prop, just a penis for the women to play with. Sometimes you don't even get to see the men's heads or faces. Blake's films play themselves out like long, fluid music videos, and though the actual orgasms of the women are in question—it seems like they never actually have an orgasm—watching them writhe, lick, and masturbate is quite enjoyable. Light fetish and kink run throughout several of his films, as do themes of master/slave lesbian entanglements, though the plot is seldom thick in any way. His films can be a great starting point for those new to porn, as they combine taste, beauty, and often light sex to create easy-on-the-eyes, sexy art films. Many of his all-girl films contain little actual sex, sometimes no anal sex, and scant cunnilingus. All of Blake's films have extremely high production values and are shot directly on film.

Seymore Butts, aka Adam Glasser (gonzo)

Whatever feelings you have about the practice of fisting, put them aside for a moment to meet Adam Glasser. A handsome man with sparkling eyes and a hidden, caustic wit, Glasser is also well known by the juvenile moniker Seymore Butts, a maker of adult films. Glasser's companies Seymore, Inc., and Big Brown Eyes, Inc. (BBE), are homespun operations, with his seventy-year-old mother employed as the accountant in their San

Fernando Valley offices. His films are a cut above most; Glasser takes pride in the work he does, going on what turns his actors on.

In December 2000, the Los Angeles Police Department (LAPD) sent its finest on a raid of Glasser's offices, looking for *Tampa Tushy Fest Part 1,* a tape Glasser made in 1999. In the raid, they confiscated the master and all copies of the tape. They later charged Glasser, his company, and his mother with one count of trafficking in obscene materials each as well as one count each of promoting the distribution of obscene materials.

People make piles of porn in Southern California every day. The powers-that-be often want to crack down on porn. So what got the boys in blue fired up enough to stage a prohibition-style raid, charge someone's accountant mom (who has nothing to do with the videos and says that porn actors are "just nice people"), and begin what would be L.A.'s first obscenity trial in eight years? *Tampa Tushy Fest Part 1* also happened to be an *Adult Video News* award-winning tape, winning "Best All-Girl Sex Scene 2000" for a hot encounter between major porn stars Alisha Klass and Chloe. It was this very scene that gave the L.A. City Attorney's office fuel to attempt a crackdown on Glasser and others like him.

The scene in question is a fisting scene, and fisting is a sex act mentioned on a 1981 memorandum listing acts the City Attorney considers to be "triggers" for obscenity charges, along with urination and female ejaculation. Fisting isn't illegal in California, and as a sexual practice is becoming more widespread as people are becoming more willing to explore their sexuality—the publication and sales of the fisting guide *Hand in the Bush* by Deborah Addington show us exactly this.

As Chloe said about fisting and the scene in *Tushy Fest:* "For me, it's almost a spiritual act. And in this particular scene, you can see that Alisha and I are having a very good time." Glasser commented on his motivations for including the controversial scene in the first place, saying: "I didn't do this fisting just to create a stir. I didn't do it because I wanted to create this controversy. I did it because I asked Chloe, 'What gets you off?' She said, 'I like it when somebody fists me.' It was so innocent! So I wanted to shoot it, and that was the reality of it.... Something that causes somebody to have eyes-rolled-in-the-back-of-their-head orgasms, that's

Fisting? Yikes!

WHEN SOMEONE IS FISTED, whether vaginally or anally, they receive penetration from their partner's entire hand, curled into a flexible, compact fist. For people who've never even contemplated penetration with larger objects, this sounds like it might hurt, and the term fisting makes it sound almost violent, as if there was punching involved. There isn't—and fisting, when done correctly with someone who likes it, doesn't hurt. In fact, for people who love the feeling of being "filled up," it can induce mind-blowing orgasms. This is exactly what it does for adult star Chloe—just watch her in any movie and you'll see one intense, authentic orgasm after another as she is penetrated by big dildos. There's no faking the pleasure she feels.

It's a very slow process that involves a lot of patience, a highly sexually aroused recipient, and a lot of lube. The person being fisted directs the action, instructing the penetrator as they go along, telling them to add a finger, add rhythm, add lube, slow down, stop, or continue. The effect is a feeling of fullness or stretching, and since both the vaginal canal and the anal canal are elastic, they do not get "stretched out," and return to their previous size soon after orgasm.

the kind of stuff that I want to see, and I think the people out there want to see it as well."

Anyone who is a consenting adult can self-determine sexual pleasure—as long as it isn't against the law. Still, the Los Angeles City Attorney's office decided to push forward with the obscenity trial. Some folks think that the prosecutors wanted to make an "example" of Glasser—though scuttlebutt suggests that the city is hoping to get federal bucks from the Bush administration if it starts cracking down on pornographers.

The goal of the City Attorney's office was a guilty charge—and they charged Glasser's mother as leverage to try to force a guilty plea from him. Prosecutors offered Glasser a deal in which he would plead guilty to obscenity, pay $1,000, and get a couple of years of probation. (The stiffest penalty for an obscenity rap is six months in the pen and a $1,000 fine.) In exchange, charges against his mother and his company would be dropped. But authorities didn't plan on the unexpected: Glasser fought back. "Why should I plead guilty? I didn't do anything wrong. Plus, this is how I put food on the table, and someone's saying I'm a criminal for it? Two women of consenting age enjoying themselves before a willing adult audience is not obscene."

On March 20, 2001, Adam Glasser walked out of the courtroom completely freed of all obscenity charges against himself, his mother Lila Glasser, and his companies in what has to be one of the best plea bargains ever reached in a local obscenity case. Glasser's company, BBE, Inc., would plead "no contest" to a charge of "creating a public nuisance" and would pay a fine of $1,000 into a "victim's restitution" fund. The company was not put on probation. All other charges against Adam Glasser, Lila Glasser, and Glasser's two companies were dropped.

"Let's be honest," Glasser said. "The $1,000 'donation,' the 'public nuisance' plea, that's really a compromise, a face-saving political move for the City Attorney's office, who didn't want to come away from this case with absolutely nothing. The charge is meaningless, and as far as I know, there have been no 'victims' of *Tampa Tushy Fest*." Glasser agreed to make all customers of *Tampa Tushy Fest* aware that a "non-fisting" version of the tape exists if they wish to purchase it, or exchange a currently owned "fisting" version for it. Otherwise, Glasser is free to sell the fisting version of *Tushy Fest* in California, safe from any charge of obscenity.

"I have been told that the list, that 1981 memorandum, is being reviewed very seriously by [L.A. City Attorney] Mr. Delgadillo and his staff," Glasser stated afterward. "I believe that they want to put their regime's own stamp on how the city handles these obscenity cases. They want to re-create the guidelines, so to speak, and from what I hear, fisting is one of the acts that is going to be reviewed because of its touch on every group of sexually active people: heterosexuals, lesbian women, and gay men. That act is pervasive among all three, and I think with all the information we provided to them, I think they became suddenly aware—I don't think they knew there were books written on fisting, and that so many websites had information available on fisting. I don't think they were aware of what's happened in this world, sexually, since 1981." Or maybe longer even longer than that, Adam.

I really like Adam Glasser's porn, for many reasons. It's basically like his own home movies, except that his friends are all in the porn business and like to have sex a lot. So the viewer gets the vicarious thrill ride of unscripted, off-the-cuff sex (the trademark of gonzo porn), but with seasoned sex performers who are having sex because they want to—not because they have to. At least that's what it feels like: porn stars letting their hair down. Lots of real female orgasms, sex with a healthy sense of fun, and the occasional joy of women penetrating the guys (and making them come like firehoses). If you don't mind the in-between scenes of Adam's shoegazing camera while he's on the phone, they're great masturbation material. And Glasser is smart, and quite witty, which reminds you that your porn is coming from someone who has a brain—something that's important to me, anyway.

Ben Dover (gonzo)

With sparkling eyes and British charm, director Ben Dover rules the English gonzo scene with a well-lubed fist. Dover got his start as a performer in 1992, appearing in a few English porn films. He took a break for three years, then, inspired by John "Buttman" Stagliano's gonzo videos, reinvented himself as Ben Dover, creating his own line of British-based gonzo/pro-am tapes. With his hand-held camera, eager libido, and trusty, always-horny male sidekicks, he elicits fun and enjoyable sexual antics from women all over England. He talks to the viewer a little, but mostly talks to the performers—though they often get so worked up and horny they don't always listen to him. The banter and humor is enough to make these films notable, but his cast of amateur, extremely sexually eager women are the real stars of this show. What's more, the people are real, unpackaged folks, so you can expect the unexpected with every tape. All types of women, a big age range, diverse bodies—you'll see shaved and hirsute, all on the same tape—and a range of motivations make each experience with each performer exciting. The action is unscripted, and anything goes, so you can always expect plenty of oral sex, toys, vaginal and anal sex, and in all the standard hetero combinations. His *British Housewife Fantasies* go to real housewives' houses for afternoons of uninhibited sex, probably one of the only "wives" series that can make the authenticity claim.

Joe Gallant (wall-to-wall/gonzo)

Maverick New York artist and filmmaker Joe Gallant is an independent porn auteur who creates porn unlike anyone else in the business. His contextualizing of porn within the framework of conceptual art is a vital contribution to the landscape of pornography. With a very artistic approach and creative visual style, he communicates in a whole different filmic language than the rest of his counterparts. He has a flair for atmosphere but invites the viewer to create their own narration to the video, filming and editing together industrial New York visuals, hand-made credits, hard-core scenes of amateur New York women having sex in all its unmade, non-porn-industry glory, scenes of his performers taking paint enemas on the sly in public, exhibitionist women in the midst of riot police, and much more. It's straight-up sex, usually safe sex, and with no music, overly made-up starlets, or any of the trappings of packaged porn. Gallant's films range from the all-sex video described above to intense fetish films depicting lots of paint enemas, and even go as far as defecation footage—check the box cover to see what you're in for. His films are not for beginners.

Jules Jordan (gonzo, wall-to-wall)

Young, blond, blue-eyed Jules Jordan entered the world of porn as an adult store manager on the East Coast. He shot a number of films before moving to California, where he was quickly noticed by John Stagliano and signed up to make films for Evil Angel Video, with Stagliano, John Leslie, and others. His films are well-shot and edited, with no music and with good lighting. They are very basic: Pretty young women (often just 18) have raunchy sex with one to four men. The men are forceful, folding, bending, and positioning the women around any way that pleases them, and the women happily comply. These films don't focus on female pleasure by any means, but the women seem to be enjoying the sex and this genre fulfills many fantasies about women being used as a sex toy for multiple male partners. The sex is never safe—that interferes with Jordan's porn ideals—and there are a lot of DPs, DVs, and DAs. Forceful, raw, nasty, and really intense—the performers can't hold back their need to throw a really nasty fuck—these films are not for everyone. Sometimes Jordan himself gets into the action, and his smooth, gentle voice and commentary adds an interesting layer to the intensity.

John Leslie (wall-to-wall/gonzo)

What could be the highest quality all-sex film you could imagine? It would likely be a John Leslie film. Beautiful and graceful all-natural women, good-looking men, blistering chemistry between the very fervent sex partners—and that's just the caliber of the performers. Mastering the art of the subtle (and well-placed not-so-subtle) camera angle, using only natural lighting or understated indoor lighting, omitting music unless it's faint jazz in the background, and often forgoing dialogue altogether, his all-sex films are the masturbation material of choice for sophisticated masturbators around the world. Blow jobs and anal sex never looked so good, and the stunning women, who have ample behinds, have a really good time. His all-sex films earn my highest ratings. You'll see plenty of threesomes, anal sex, blow jobs, and double penetrations in a Leslie film, and condom use is on-again, off-again.

Leslie no longer appears in front of the camera, but when he did he was one of the consummate actors of his day. Handsome, leading-man material, Leslie could really act and put passion and fiery desire into each of his Golden Age performances. He was born and raised in the Midwest and worked at an Ohio steel mill in the late 1950s. The lure of the New York art scene found him in the Big Apple in the early 1960s, where he hoped to become a painter. Like most artists, things didn't work out as planned for Leslie and he ended up working in New York's then-thriving underground magazine market as an illustrator. He got into the early 1970s swinging scene and also found side work as a blues harmonica player.

He moved to San Francisco in 1974, where he met people working in the fledgling hard-core film industry. His charisma and casual sex appeal caused his friends to urge him to try his hand at adult performing. He became one of the most popular male performers of the late '70s and throughout the '80s, always turning in sensual and erotic work. His fine acting skills helped him land meaty roles in lots of top-notch productions and he's won just about every industry award there is for performers. He moved behind the cameras in the mid-'80s, one of the first men to make the now-common transition from performer to director.

Sean Michaels (wall-to-wall, features)

Tall, unapologetically attractive Sean Michaels is the ultimate ladies' man, and an icon to his male fans. He's a hardworking African-American male actor who has run up against racism in the adult industry and has overcome it by turning the camera around and making porn with what he calls "no color lines." Michaels has been a major force in changing the face and attitudes of the adult industry toward black performers. The racism in the industry surfaced, in his case, when some white actresses refused to work with him as a black actor. Squeamish directors who were afraid to portray interracial sex—and possibly fearing legal problems in racist communities—have also edited him out of several videos.

Michaels was born Andre Allen in Brooklyn, New York. He moved out west in 1989, and quickly began his porn career. His above-average acting skills enabled him to land roles that hadn't previously gone to black actors. He's a gentle-spirited, lanky, chiseled man with a sly, sweet grin that lets you know he's having the time of his life with the women he's playing with, and loving every minute of it. His boyish good looks have proven to be irresistible to starlets and female fans for over a decade, and he's still going strong on both sides of the camera with his production company, Sean Michaels Productions. The star of more than 700 hard-core features and now one of the most earnest directors in the biz, Michaels is deservedly the most famous black man to ever appear in porn. He's a member of the *AVN* Hall of Fame and a two-time winner of the Fans of X-Rated Entertainment Male Favorite Award, and continues to win awards every year.

Sean Michaels' efforts as a producer and director have kept him at the forefront of black-themed and interracial videos. His all-sex films include pairs of attractive men and women who are clearly into each other, having great sex. The *Naughty Wives Club* series has gorgeous women having a blast getting it on with guys (and sometimes each other), and the occasional curvaceous unaltered body is refreshing and exciting. The production values aren't high—often a single room or location and static lighting—but the enthusiasm is. There is always a scene with Michaels himself having his trademark turgid, tender sex with one of the starlets, and his *Special Auditions* series is all Sean Michaels and the women. Sometimes there is music, and sometimes not.

Jewel D'Nyle (wall-to-wall)

Hypersexual and smart as a whip, brunette Jewel D'Nyle came from Colorado and turned heads the minute she debuted in adult, circa 1998. Jewel is dedicated to improving the adult industry, and feels a responsibility to promote the growing trend toward bigger and better productions, with skilled acting professionals. She wants to see more erotic entertainment that features better-directed talent, in high-caliber scripts. Jewel feels the future of the adult industry "lies in achieving legitimacy and respect approaching that currently enjoyed by mainstream entertainment." She directs and stars in her fun-loving, all-sex series, *Babes in Pornland*.

Ed Powers (gonzo)

This former New Yorker was one of the men who single-handedly pioneered the "gonzo" genre. Armed with a video camera and nothing more, he would talk to women interested in performing sex on camera and they would do so, having their first-time onscreen sex with Ed. He has become the "everyman" of porn; he is not conventionally attractive, is older, has a receding hairline, wears glasses, and shows that you don't have to look a certain way to have heated sex with beautiful women.

His *Dirty Debutantes* series is his most famous (and lengthy) work, the debutantes being women who have never had on-camera sex, though many are strippers and exhibitionists in their own right. In the same settings on a single tape, he'll talk to the women as they sit in front of the camera, making them laugh and tell about themselves, and as they begin to play with themselves, Ed keeps the banter going as they both get progressively turned on, and Ed joins in to have sex with his subject. And did I mention that Ed is a total goofball? There is a clear spirit of fun here, the women have a really good time—they often orgasm—and each pairing employs safer sex gear. Ed feels that condoms are respectful and smart, and even puts condoms on shared sex toys. His series are excellent, with no rough stuff, and his couples series, *Porn O Plenty,* is especially fun. He does not use music in his videos.

Shane (gonzo/wall-to-wall)

Shane rocks! Cute, curvy, and exuding an all-American-girl freshness, blonde and busty Shane looks like she'd be the chick that just blew by you on a snowboard, or the kind of gal every skater or BMX-er would want as his hottie girlfriend. But Shane's got two things on her mind— having lots of fun and having lots of hot sex. She started out in porn as gonzo filmmaker Seymore Butts's (Adam Glasser's) girlfriend, and together in the mid-'90s they made porn that packed in so much chemistry between them, you'd almost have to wear a biohazard suit to watch it and avoid a total meltdown. *Shane on the Loose* and *Seymore Butts Goes Nuts* are great examples of the young, attractive couple in lust. Since their breakup, Shane has taken matters into her own hands, directing and star-ring in her own series of female-gonzo films, cruising the U.S. in a mobile home that's got to be the happiest RV in existence. Her many delectable series feature gorgeous gals who love sex and have a hot time having it— and fans of "reality TV" will enjoy the girl with a camera who follows her friends around and eggs them on with their sexual exploits.

Shane approaches her genre from a number of angles; in her *Slumber Party* series she gets groups of starlets and pals together for an evening or a weekend of partying and having lots of hot girl–girl sex. In other series, she'll get groups of men and women together for weekends at a river vacation, or just film a bunch of guys and gals having sex all over a house. There is a college-guy and -girl feel to the cast and the flavor of

Pimp and Circumstance:
Snoop Dogg and the Hip-Hop/Porn Connection

HIP-HOP HAS LONG FLIRTED with porn in music videos and lyric content, and in 2001 the relationship became big news with rapper Snoop Dogg's unifying marriage of hip-hop and porn with his *Hustler* release, *Snoop Dogg's Doggystyle*. In a smart cross-selling move the video was released with eleven original songs by Dogg combined with hard-core sex scenes, appealing to his fans and helping to push more units out the door. The tape sold widely, and Snoop continues to appear in porn under *Hustler's* banner. As in *Doggystyle*, he doesn't perform or direct but still helms the action, introducing scenes with pearls of wisdom about "his bitches" and "breaking them in," and posing as a Don Juan kind of pimp in *Diary of a Pimp*. Fortunately, like any pimp, he refers to his human property as little girls that he has saved and works really hard to take care of—and you can see in the films that they're now free from the shackles of identity and personality and don't have to worry about those bother-some orgasms any more because no one gives a shit about women getting off in these films. However, the biggest crime onscreen is the fact that the videos are unremarkable save for the fact that Dogg is a celebrity and Mr. Marcus performs in them; without women coming in them, it's pretty boring porn. Although others will want to claw their eyes out when they see the editing of the sex scenes.... Hip-hop and porn continue their marriage, with Ice-T directing and starring in *Pimpin' 101*, a pseudo how-to guide based on his past as a pimp. DJ Yella (NWA) has been involved in porn since the mid-'90s, long before Snoop Dogg stepped up to the plate. Too $hort has signed up with production powerhouse Adam and Eve to create a line of videos that feature the rapper performing in the videos and original soundtracks by the artist, And many crossover female hip-hop and rap performers such as India, Heather Hunter, and Chaos have joined the parade.

the couplings, and many of the performers have tattoos and piercings, look like an MTV spring-break crowd, and definitely appeal to the snowboarding and skate crowds. No music, just natural sound; the sex is hot, hot, hot; and the fresh faces are exciting.

Rocco Siffredi (gonzo, wall-to-wall)

It's easy to see why Rocco Siffredi has so many fans, both male and female, when you watch him go absolutely crazy with lust for his beautiful European female sex partners. One of the most popular male performers today, Siffredi is an Italian who appears in videos from around the world, and has his own line of videos. Handsome and with great acting skills, he has performed roles ranging from bespectacled geek and muscleman to the Marquis De Sade and a self-parodying porn actor. He has an enormous female fan following, and it's not just for his big package—his genuine affection for his onscreen lovers is riveting, and he can even convey that affection when he's playing rough. And play rough he certainly does, with style and intensity. He holds and coos, kisses and makes much eye contact, while he genuinely goes crazy with lust and reverence for his female performers, while simultaneously he face-slaps, spits on genitals and in mouths, pulls costars' heads onto his cock while they choke, spanks, forces hands and feet into their mouths, and more.

Rocco Siffredi got into European porn in the mid-'80s, but it was his performances in a string of Buttman flicks in the early '90s that brought him to the attention of American fans. He played John Stagliano's sidekick in quite a few of the hottest Buttman features, showing off his super-charged sexuality to a receptive American audience. Some of his best work can be found in *Buttman's European Vacation 1*.

Recently, Siffredi's been producing and directing his own line of features for Evil Angel, all of which are packed with his signature nasty antics. The raw camera style in his all-sex films adds to the immediacy of the sex, the lighting is never distracting, there is no music (except Europop in the introductions), and everything is shot in Europe, typically Italy, so the locations are unusual and the commentary and dialogue are in another language, though sometimes in halting English—all of which makes his films a refreshing break from California porn. Not to mention that the European women look like very real, very pretty girls, the kind you'd meet on a regular day, and not the overly packaged starlets or trashy blondes in American porn. His camera is often hand-held and the shots are sometimes weaving and unsteady, and his production values can be rough or high, depending on the series.

John "Buttman" Stagliano (gonzo, features)

With John Stagliano, it's all about the booty: beautiful, lush, buoyant, bouncing, round, and enthusiastic booty. If you like backsides, anal sex in all its permutations, and women who like it too, any film by Buttman is a gold mine. And though he shoots in a gonzo style, consciously part of the action as both cameraman and director of the action, unlike other gonzo auteurs his tapes have high production values and great quality all around. He's known for interesting locations (sometimes shot in Europe), terrific lighting, no music, excellent camera work, respectful interactions, and gorgeous performers who really want to be there—and are totally enjoying the sex. It's easy to see why his work is so highly regarded, and legendary.

Born in Chicago in the early 1950s, Stagliano intended to pursue economics and moved to Southern California in the early '70s to go to school, but picked up jobs for extra cash as a nude model. By 1979 he was a Chippendale's dancer (can you imagine Chippendale's parties in the late '70s? Whoa). At any rate, by 1983 he was involved in porn, and produced videos with Bruce Seven until 1989, when he formed Evil Angel Video with Patrick Collins. The name for what is now his sprawling video empire came from his old stripping name, Evil John, and a former girlfriend, Angel.

The *Adventures of Buttman* was released in 1989, changing the face of porn forever with the introduction of gonzo-style shooting, along with Ed Powers' *Dirty Debutantes*. These no-plot, all-sex, "horny guy with a camera" adventures were groundbreaking and well received, and over the years Stagliano refined his fun-loving, butt-grabbing Buttman persona and his own filmic style.

Stagliano performed in his videos until he contracted HIV, when he retired from filmmaking and openly announced his condition, and his life has become an open book for the industry, which you can see in *Buttman Confidential,* where he talks openly about his sexual risk-taking, contracting HIV, working in the business, and his outlook. Recently, and fortunately for us, Stagliano has returned behind the camera to direct more Buttman videos, turning out his highest quality work ever. His newer work has high production values, is well-thought-out (though still unscripted and improvised), and frames the scenes cleverly. He features lots of anal, some gaping, often intense chemistry between performers (some even feature real-life porn couples, such as Jazmine and Nacho Vidal), though he leaves safer-sex choices to the performers—making condom use rarely evident. He also directs features, which may be some of his most mind-blowing work to date, creating feature epics that in look, feel, and screenwriting appear just like a big-budget Hollywood film, though they focus on sexually frustrated characters and contain (sometimes literally) hours of sex.

Randy West (gonzo)

For twenty years Randy West was a performer, and a favorite sex partner of Ashlyn Gere until he picked up a camera in the mid-'90s to film gonzo style, pro-am videos in his trademark series, *Up N Cummers*. One of the first purposefully pro-am series, it was a huge hit and became the vehicle of choice for starlets who wanted to get noticed. In #11, he captured a new, unenhanced Jenna Jameson; #40 saw Raylene get her start; and #73 featured a fresh Tera Patrick. With well over a hundred in the series, it's a great archive for porn star entries and good to watch for fresh, enthusiastic talent.

His production values are minimal, as typically he shoots his scenes in one or two rooms of a house. The women talk to Randy as he's behind the camera, while he chides them, encourages them, and is full of admiration for the female form, which shows in both banter and camerawork. Then the women undress and have sex with Randy, or a man that they prefer—and sometimes the viewer is treated to starlets and their real-life loving husbands or boyfriends. The ejaculations are both internal and external. No two films have the exact same formula—some have more of one sex act than another, or an extra such as outdoor urination (nonsexual). He also directed *Real Female Masturbation*.

All-Sex Video Reviews

This genre is enormous—it would be impossible to cover every single series and tape. Instead, what follows is a handpicked selection of highlights that feature the very best in quality, and a wide-ranging sample of what's available, with suggested favorite series. Quite a few of these series, as well as individual tapes, have won awards. Use this as a starting point for your explorations.

Amateur Angels series

Cute girls showcase girl-next-door charm and have first-time experiences on camera, though usually the women have had onscreen sex once or twice before. But their freshness is startling and their experiences are genuine, and many tapes feature the women with either their real-life boyfriends or an established male performer. Wylder directs the action gonzo-style, and the performers are having a smiley, great time.

DIRECTOR: Luc Wylder, series began in 2001.

Babes Ballin' Boys series

In this series, whose quality ranges from couplings with great chemistry to scenes with bad sound and unenthused performers, women wear strap-on dildos and bend the boys over for a whole lot of backdoor fun. When the scenes are hot, they're mind-blowing, and the men have huge hard-ons while the smiling, sexy women give it to them. Look for tapes that have scenes with stars such as sexy Tina Tyler and you'll have a great pick; but either way the men in this series really like anal penetration from lovely ladies, and strap-on sex is only part of the sex acts the pairings perform.

DIRECTOR: Various, series started in 1997.

Dominant Women	Violet's Top Choice	Intense Chemistry	Extreme Sex Acts	Great for Newbies

(Jewel D'Nyle's) Babes in Pornland series

Performer Jewel D'Nyle is known for her nastiness, and she directs and performs like a pro in this excellent series of title-themed releases. She pairs exciting starlets with established male performers, turning out many highly regarded and critically praised sex scenes. The camera angles, editing, clarity of images, and color saturation make for mesmerizing scenes, while the women tease and taunt before throwing themselves into each sex scene with abandon.

DIRECTOR: Jewel D'Nyle, series started in 2001.

Teen Babes, Anal Babes, All-American Babes, Asian Babes, Busty Babes, Interracial Babes, Latin Babes (and more)

Barely Legal series

Hustler's series of hit-or-miss performances featuring women who are 18 (or are supposed to be, anyway—likely they are older). They look young and wear teen accessories, and have sex with male porn performers. Some have minimal plots, usually about a young girl getting men to have sex with her—like, wow, that's new. Anyway, good for folks with young teenage girl fantasies.

DIRECTOR: Various; series began in 1987.

Bend Over Boyfriend 2: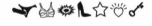
More Rockin', Less Talkin'

Not a sequel to the educational film *Bend Over Boyfriend* but a continuation of the theme by the same directors. Real-life Gen-X couples (and a real-life trio) perform unscripted vignettes where the outcome is the boyfriend (or husband) being penetrated by a beautiful woman with a strap-on—with orgasms for all. Excellent lighting and camerawork, and terrific chemistry between the amateur couples who are sexually experienced, making the sex on this tape superior to most other male anal penetration videos. Each scene has a nice, unrushed feel and is lightly kinky, with fantasy themes including cop and prostitute, white trash couple, mistress and ponyboy, and more. Read more about SIR Video in Chapter 10, "Lesbian, All-Girl, Bisexual, and Gay Features."

DIRECTOR: Shar Rednour and Jackie Strano (SIR Video), 1999, 80 min.

CAST: Chloe, Dr. Carol Queen, Daphne, Mistress Olive, Topper Felix, Butch, Scott Blue, Troy Trixx, others

NOTE: Independent filmmaker.

Woman Penetrates Man	Natural Cast	Unsightly Boob Job	Well-Made Film	Real Female Orgasm

Andrew Blake films

Sumptuous, sensuous, high-gloss, and high-class, the top erotic models who pop-ulate Blake's films are some of the most amazing sexual creatures on earth, and with music overlaying the action, they engage in scenes that are unbelievably decadent and outrageous. Usually one woman will be dominant, making her other sexy femme, female slaves lick her high heels, service her male studs (who are literally no more than a sex toy), or sit still while she eats her dinner from their quivering bodies, reclining atop a carefully set table. You'll see all kinds of light femme-on-femme BDSM, including candle wax, spanking, leashes, and nipple clamps. No expense is spared, and the productions are filmed in mansions on location in Europe and costumed lavishly with everything from period Victorian outfits to mind-blowing rubber gear. You seldom even see the men's faces as the women take their time extracting every drop of pleasure. However, the women usually take center stage together or masturbating solo, and while they look like they're getting really worked up, they never seem to have an orgasm. Some of Blake's films have a minimal plot, and some are just long, languid scenes of pol-ished sensuality. It's erotic eye candy in its highest form. All Blake videos are shot on film, and it should be noted that the music accompanying the women's mas-turbation and gyrations isn't for everyone, though it is from composer Raoul Valve. The following titles are a sample of Blake's oeuvre.

NOTE: Filmed in Europe, shot on film.

Aria, 2000, 81 min.
A lingering tribute to female eroticism via the sexual attentions between two women who lick, paddle, and restrain each other, with every inch of skin wor-shipped. Has a male–female sex scene and stars curvaceous Aria Giovanni.

Blond and Brunettes, 2001, 95 min.
Anita Blond and Aria Giovanni are blonde and brunette, meeting up with some of the world's finest centerfolds for displays of their wealthy and mildly kinky lifestyles. Has a tribal/techno score, won an *AVN* award.

Captured Beauty, 1995, 78 min.
Penthouse Pet Dahlia Grey and a lot of all-girl, no-penetration BDSM.

Dark Angel, 1994, 115 min.
In a sequel to *Paris Chic,* Dahlia Grey is submissive to a cruel mistress in this docu-drama about Dahlia's rise to erotic stardom.

Dominant Women

Violet's Top Choice

Intense Chemistry

Extreme Sex Acts

Great for Newbies

Delirious, 1998, 118 min.
Dahlia Grey is a French heiress who subjects her cousin to sexual temptations and irresistible betrayals, making the cousin's boyfriend into a sex slave.

Desire, 1994, 85 min.
Zara Whites is an art gallery owner with many gallery-based sexual fantasies.

Girlfriends, 2001, 99 min.
Leg and foot worship are taken to dizzying heights, with mild BDSM and a good ambient sound track. Features Aria Giovanni, Justine, and others.

Hidden Obsessions, 1993, 90 min.
Janine stars in her first erotic film playing a writer who decides to live out fantasies instead of writing them. Features a famous ice dildo scene, and won three *AVN* awards.

High Heels, 1998, 90 min.
Models from the pages of *Penthouse, Perfect 10,* and *Legshow* frolic in Italy playing dominance and submission games, featuring lots of leg shots, lingerie, public exhibitionism, and high heels. Won an *AVN* award in 1998.

House of Dreams, 1990, 76 min.
A Blake classic starring Zara White, who wanders through a dream house having lightly kinky fantasies. Won four *AVN* awards; also features Ashlyn Gere, Jeanna Fine, Raven, Rocco Siffredi, and Randy Spears.

Justine, 2003, 102 min.
Andrew Blake's photography studio is the setting for beautiful Justine and her playmates to dress in sexy lingerie and engage in girl–girl fantasies that include hot wax, a glass dildo, and a fanny swatter.

Les Femmes Erotiques, 1993, 120 min.
Julia Ann is featured in one of her earliest films that centers on virtual reality trips to sexual fantasy scenarios, from the Roaring Twenties to fun in the stables. A large number of male–female scenes, and a whopping fourteen sex scenes total.

Paris Chic, 1997, 92 min.
Lea Martini and Anita Blond shine as an erotic photographer and a young model who become entwined in a dominant–submissive relationship.

Pin-Ups, 1999, 120 min.
Dahlia Grey stars in a plot-free film that has lots of masturbation and girl–girl encounters.

Woman Penetrates Man   Natural Cast   Unsightly Boob Job   Well-Made Film   Real Female Orgasm

Pin-Ups 2, 2000, 90 min.
Retro beauty Dita is featured with Anita Blond and Inari Vachs in this stunning film that is a series of scenes with no plot whatsoever.

Playthings, 1998, 110 min.
Dahlia Grey and her beautiful playthings cavort and tease within the world of nude modeling, with a focus on legs and breasts. Won an *AVN* award in 1998.

Secret Paris, 2000, 90 min.
More beautiful women in wall-to-wall modeling, masturbation, and girl–girl scenes, with one male–female sex scene.

Secrets, 1990, 80 min.
Ashlyn Gere stars as a Hollywood madam in this early Blake film, which is a critics' favorite and contains many male–female sex scenes. Stars Gere, Zara Whites, Rocco Siffredi, Jeanna Fine, and others.

Unleashed, 1996, 86 min.
Asia Carrera featured with Dahlia Grey in this film where a magic pendant makes the fantasies of two women come true.

Black Booty Cam series

With an accent on anals and facials, as well as big beautiful butts, this is an all-black, all-sex series. They usually contain natural women, bare-bones production values, and lots of sex with enthusiastic black male and female performers. A few were shot on location in Brazil, with all-Brazilian cast members, and many feature first-time performers. As with most porn, some scenes fall flat, while others shine.
DIRECTOR: Various, series started in 2000.

Blowjob Fantasies series

One wet, slurpy blow job scene after another is all you get on these tapes, with numerous porn star appearances. Quality varies widely from scene to scene: One scene will be excellent, the next utterly abysmal. For fans of blow jobs it's a decent choice, especially with all the expert sword swallowers on each tape. Facial come shots for all. Higher quality can be found in *Voyeur's Favorites: Blowjobs and Anals* (dir. John Leslie).
DIRECTOR: Various, series started in 1998.

Dominant Women	Violet's Top Choice	Intense Chemistry	Extreme Sex Acts	Great for Newbies

Boss Bitches series

This series is very hit-or-miss, with cut-rate production values, though occasionally the scenes are gems. Women dominate the men, bossing them around, shaving them, and strapping it on and penetrating them. The women are not dominatrixes, and many are trying strap-on sex for the first time, so often the scenes are too rushed or half-hearted. But sometimes they're worth the effort, so especially look for tapes that feature recognizable names, such as Tina Tyler.

DIRECTOR: Henri Pachard, series started in 1999.

Buttman series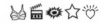

John Stagliano has taken admiration of the female backside to dizzying heights, and for anyone who likes beautiful natural gals with generous bottoms and who loves anal sex, this series is an unending supply of heaven. In his adventures, Buttman roams Europe, Brazil, and a little bit of the U.S. with his camera, filming one hot Euro babe after another who perform uninhibited, intense sex acts for the camera, with well-hung (usually European) studs. The scenes are then edited together for a particular tape. His banter with the performers is fun, respectful, enthusiastic about sex, and quite humorous, and everyone laughs and has a good time. What's nice is that the women look and enjoy the sex as mature young women, not the giggly girls usually found in typical American gonzo porn. Erotic and enjoyable in feel and atmosphere, the exquisite locales are a far cry from cheap Southern California hotel rooms. Many tapes feature Rocco Siffredi in one or more scenes. Often the women (and their men) are making their first or only appearances for the camera, and real-life couples crop up from time to time. The *Buttman* videos regularly win *AVN* awards.

DIRECTOR: John "Buttman" Stagliano

Buttman's Bend Over Babes
Big beautiful female butts and spicy European women from the U.S., Brazil, and Hungary, having lots of anal sex in all combinations. This series is a favorite; high-quality filming, exuberant performances, and torrid sex make this a very popular choice. Find more of John Stagliano's films in "Feature Films," Chapter 6.

Buttman's Big Tit Adventure
Voluptuous women with large natural breasts are the order of the day, and the tapes are location-specific, including Texas, Los Angeles, and Budapest.

Woman Penetrates Man   Natural Cast   Unsightly Boob Job   Well-Made Film   Real Female Orgasm

Buttman's Rio Carnival Hardcore/Parties

On the streets and in clubs, all during Carnival, the women turn into crazy exhibitionists and the men go wild for them. Stagliano edits together his favorite scenes, and boy, they grow those booties lush and big in Brazil!

Seymore Butts series

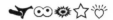

Director Seymore Butts is a pretty average young guy—except for the camera he carries with him everywhere he goes, and the porn stars and adult filmmakers he hangs out with. Butts's tapes are essentially his home movies, albeit home movies that are filmed pretty well and contain explicit sex. But unlike the stereotype of guy-with-a-camera-making-porn, he's charming and likeable, funny and genuine, and he manages to capture something that the others don't—porn performers having relaxed, enjoyable, and very heated sex. His tapes are informal, genuine, and full of incredible orgasms. You'll see women coming in all manner of ways, and gushing orgasms are not rare. There's lots of anal sex, oral sex (controlled by the women, no "forcing"—and he captures some of the hottest blow jobs anywhere in porn) and group scenes. Butts made quite a few tapes with his ex-girlfriend Shane (her films follow in this chapter), and those sing with the chemistry of two people in love; some of his tapes include another former girlfriend, porn star Taylor Hayes, and their adventures are great to watch, too. In the Shane videos, Seymore is being sent explicit fan mail in the form of a videotape made by a sexy mystery girl, who turns out to be Shane, and then the video progresses on their adventures together (and no, they're not monogamous). With Butts's videos, the budgets aren't huge, the camera sometimes moves about drunkenly, and sometimes "reality TV" lagtime ensues as Butts moves through his life from one sex scene to the next, but the wait is always worth it. The pros think so too, since his series wins countless *AVN* awards. For a Seymore Butts plot-driven feature, see *Dinner Party 2: The Buffet* in Chapter 6, "Feature Films."

DIRECTOR: Seymore Butts, aka Adam Glasser

Seymore Butts and His Mystery Girl, 1994, 120 min.

We watch some of the tape from the nasty masturbator (the mystery girl), then Butts goes about his business setting up his pal Rocco Siffredi to have sex with two women, and the tape goes on into one hot sex scene after another.

CAST: Shane, Danyel Cheeks, Tracy Prince, Sierra, Rocco Siffredi, Butch, TT Boy

Dominant Women

Violet's Top Choice

Intense Chemistry

Extreme Sex Acts

Great for Newbies

Seymore Butts Bustin Out My Best, 1995, 140 min.

If all you want to see is nonstop sex shot by Butts, with plenty of female orgasms, this compilation tape fits the bill.

CAST: Yvonne, Alex Jordan, Sierra, Danyel Cheeks, Alicia Rio, Jazzmine, Jessica Fox, Celeste, Lacey Rose, Shane, Rebeca Barbot, Sheila Stome, Laurel Canyon, Brandy Alexander, Devin

Seymore Butts in Paradise, 1994, 120 min.

Seymore finally meets the mystery girl, his then-real-life lover, Shane. They run away to Mexico, where they parasail, pick up strippers, and have really fiery, passionate sex.

CAST: Shane, Devon, Nina, Ron Jeremy, Paree, Seymore Butts

Seymore Butts Meets the Tushy Girls, 1997, 140 min.

This is a sequel, but never mind the beginning.... This tape shows Seymore making then-newcomer Alisha Klass's sexual fantasy come true, then taking her to meet his porn star friends so she can get acquainted with folks in the biz—*really* acquainted. Lots of anal sex, including a scene with male anal penetration.

CAST: Alisha Klass, Samantha Stylle, Seymore Butts, Mark Davis, Shanna McCullough, Dave Hardman, TT Boy, Tom Byron

Chica Boom series

This award-winning series features lovely feminine Latinas having honest, delicious, slippery sex with each other and well-hung men. Women from Mexico, Italy, Peru, Puerto Rico, and more team up with male porn stars for hours of vignettes that contain teasing, passionate, hard-driving sex. While not much was spent on sets, it's a well-shot sted in 2001; won *AVN* awards in 2000, 2002 for Best Ethnic Series.

Woman Penetrates Man

Natural Cast

Unsightly Boob Job

Well-Made Film

Real Female Orgasm

Chloe's gonzo titles

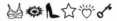

The porn starlet known for her beauty, natural figure, and arresting, authentic orgasms took to the director's chair and started making all-sex films of her own. Chloe's films have very basic production values, and some tapes have sound issues, but they burn up the screen with incendiary sex. She commands incredible, focused sex from her performers (who are sometimes real-life couples) and jumps in front of the camera to get satisfaction and lose herself in her astounding climaxes. And that's what her videos are all about: female orgasms. They star plenty of natural beauties, such as Ava Vincent and Keisha, and they're all focused on one thing: the women getting off, for real, with well-hung sex partners who are more than happy to help. Sex acts include oral, anal, penis–vagina intercourse, and sex toys—usually big ones!

DIRECTOR: Chloe

Chloe's Acting Up, 2001, 80 min.

Chloe's Catalina Cum-Ons, 2000, 154 min.

Chloe Cums First, 2000, 80 min.

Chloe's "I Came, Did You?" 1999, 80 min.

Welcome to Chloeville 1–4, all in 2000

Christoph's Beautiful Girls

French porn star Christoph Clark has a knack for finding and filming stunning natural European beauties, and is a terrific performer himself, to boot. His hand-held gonzo-style camerawork is among the best—fluid, seamless, and hot as hell as he captures amazing sex moments between his performers on the fly, and not necessarily with the usual over/under close-ups. The performers are beautiful and they walk, talk, and move like cats. When Clark himself gets into the action, all bets are off as the sex becomes unrushed and delirious, and Clark manages to have multiple orgasms. The sex is in all permutations, without a focus on any one act.

DIRECTOR: Christoph Clark, series started in 2000, won an AVN award in 2002 for best foreign release.

NOTE: Foreign release.

| Dominant Women | Violet's Top Choice | Intense Chemistry | Extreme Sex Acts | Great for Newbies |

Deep Inside films

The series focuses on one well-known female porn star, featuring her personally selected favorite scenes. These tapes are a gold mine for chemistry-packed scenes and scenes when a starlet has an emotionally charged sexual experience, a memorable first-time encounter, or a scene where they had really, really good sex. A good place to look when you have a favorite star, want to watch a tape that might have the star with her real-life lover, or just want to see a starlet have authentic orgasms. The directors are always different, and recently the expert director Veronica Hart has been trying her hand, creating some amazing collaborative work with today's top stars. The cast centers on the featured performer: people looking for, or trying to avoid, physical features such as fake breasts should make a case-by-case assessment.

DIRECTOR: Various, series started in 1982.

SERIES STARS INCLUDE: Anna Malle (1999), Annie Sprinkle (1982), Ariana (1996), Asia Carrera (1997), Chloe (2002), Deidre Holland (1993), Ginger Lynn (1987), Jeanna Fine (1992), Jill Kelly (1997), Juli Ashton (1996), Keisha (1994), Kelly O'Dell (1993), Kylie Ireland (1999), Missy (1997), Nikita (2000), Nina Hartley 1 (1993), Nina Hartley 2 (1998), Shalya LaVeaux (1997), Shannah McCullough (1992), Tyfanny Million (1995), Vanessa Del Rio (1986), Vicca (2000)

Deep Inside Felicia

All-natural starlet Felicia explodes with authentic orgasms in every scene, and because she only does girls, it's a great collection of sizzling girl-girl scenes (though men perform with other starlets on occasion). Directed by Veronica Hart.

Deep Inside Jill Kelly

Loved by female and male fans alike, voluptuous Kelly plays opposite real-life partners, including a wedding night scene with a man whom she deeply loved at the time. Directed by Veronica Hart.

Deep Inside Kylie Ireland

Squishy, sexy Ireland excels in this star-studded title, where every nasty scene drips with chemistry between Ireland and her partners. Includes a well-filmed orgy, a sweet scene with Sean Michaels, and another with Jenna Jameson and Felicia—and whipped cream.

Woman Penetrates Man

Natural Cast

Unsightly Boob Job

Well-Made Film

Real Female Orgasm

Dirty Debutantes series

The fact that this series has reached more than 200 installments attests to the popularity of Ed Powers's bare-bones, all-amateur productions. It's just Powers and his stationary or hand-held camera filming first-timers on the bed or couch, with minimal production values. After the women chat with Powers, they undress and play with themselves, then Powers and the new performer have safe sex, with no stops or pauses. Sometimes the women team up, or have threesomes with Powers or a sidekick. However, you never know what's going to happen because the moments are unstaged. The banter is sweet and playful, the women often bring their favorite sex toys, and Powers is reverent toward the women. He's no porn stud, but instead a refreshing real, regular guy. His series has been the launching pad of choice for several of today's big-name starlets, and he's raked in the *AVN* awards.

DIRECTOR: Ed Powers

Black Dirty Debutantes

All black debs in every box!

Bus Stop Tales

His early series, where, gonzo-style, he meets and talks to the women prior to their first onscreen appearance. We hear their sexual likes and dislikes, learning about them and making the ensuing sex steam with more intimacy than the usual gonzo fare.

Deep Inside Dirty Debutantes

Previous Debs return for more scenes, though there's still a debut in each video.

More Dirty Debs

More of the same, slightly different title. #3 has a female-penetrating-male strap-on scene.

Porn O Plenty

All newcomers, with more focus on getting to know the women.

| Dominant Women | Violet's Top Choice | Intense Chemistry | Extreme Sex Acts | Great for Newbies |

Ben Dover's series

That Ben Dover is a busy Brit. With several series and numerous installments, you have to wonder if every woman in England hasn't had this guy knocking on their front (or back) door. This is English gonzo, folks, and it's done with a fun, humorous, and endearing style that showcases the smarts and wit of British women, and Dover himself, of course. He's funny, the women are cracking up and making jokes, but at the same time everyone's getting each other really turned on. The sexual heat on a Dover shoot is tangible, and after a while no one can control themselves, so Dover, his male sidekicks, and the cute, curvy gals all get it on. It's clear that everyone loves his or her job. The shooting is just man-with-a-camera and no fancy anything, the men are regular English guys (read: not porn hunks with sexy accents, just accents), and the women are refreshingly diverse in appearance. Shaved, hairy, curvy, thin—it's all here, all natural, and all in fun. He has many titles, all thematically named. See: *Cheek Mates* (all-anal), *English Muffins* (just 18 and legal), *Eager Beavers, Extremely Wild Wenches, English Porno Groupies,* and *Puttin on the Brits.* Also see his *British Housewife Fantasies*—real housewives, of all shapes and sizes, having unrehearsed sex with Dover and his boys at their houses.

DIRECTOR: Ben Dover

NOTE: Foreign release.

Gush; Oh My Gush

There's little to this series except scene after scene of women and men having enthusiastic, athletic sex in all the usual formula positions and combinations, except each scene finishes after the women come—for a change! The men do everything necessary to make each of the women female ejaculate, in sweaty scenes that involve the women calling all the shots to get off. The filming is nicely done and the chemistry is great between partners, and the men use tongues, fingers, sex toys, and their penises to stimulate the frenzied gals, with lots of extreme close-ups. *Gush* is the easier to find second series, and has slightly harder sex than *Oh My Gush.* Most, but not all, of the ejaculations are authentic.

DIRECTOR: Various; *Oh My Gush* began in 1995, *Gush* in 1999.

| Woman Penetrates Man | Natural Cast | Unsightly Boob Job | Well-Made Film | Real Female Orgasm |

Jules Jordan's Flesh Hunter series

On the "hunt for perfect specimens," Jules Jordan digs up plenty of young women who like it very, very rough. Unlike a Rocco Siffredi film where the women sometimes become exhausted by the pounding, the women in *Flesh Hunter* give it right back, creating perfect fantasies where ecstatically sexual young gals push the men to give them more. It's multiple men on one woman, or a woman receiving large anal insertions by Jordan himself. Top-quality fare for fans of submissive-female fantasies, where the women are aware of how arousing the fantasy is. High production values and great editing. Oh, and lots of anal sex.

DIRECTOR: Jules Jordan, series began in 2002.

John Leslie's series

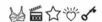

Erotic, sensual, explicit, and arousingly authentic in both heat and chemistry, John Leslie's films capture sex on camera like no others: Stunning European and American women have unbelievable sex for Leslie's camera, and he has a superior approach to the camerawork, editing, and lighting, while eliciting mind-blowing performances from male and female performers alike. Leslie seldom makes his presence obtrusive, and instead has refined his sophisticated film style as viewer-as-voyeur, making him one of the undisputed masters of his craft. Eloquent, often natural lighting, long unedited shots, no music, and fervent, insatiable performers are the hallmarks of a Leslie film. Also, his performers are very attractive: good-looking men and naturally beautiful, minimally made-up women. Quite a few starlets have had their first scenes in his films. They feature lots of incredible blow jobs, anal sex, two men and one woman, and a healthy dose of double penetrations. Because Leslie manages to capture one crucial element of supercharged, authentic sex—his performers are completely focused on each other—it's tough to miss with one of his videos.

NOTE: Foreign release.

John Leslie's Fresh Meat

The first video was a ghost story about a butcher…but the series turned into a big-butt sexfest that often features women in their first performances. Heavy focus on anal sex in most of the tapes: Read the box covers to get specifics. This series regularly takes home *AVN* awards, such as #3 (1996), #4 (1997), and #5 (1998).

Dominant Women

Violet's Top Choice

Intense Chemistry

Extreme Sex Acts

Great for Newbies

John Leslie's Voyeur

The camera is you, the viewer, as a voyeur who spies on couples and threesomes. Shots begin away from the action as the sex starts, and the camera approaches as the sex escalates. Shots sometimes come through windows, make use of sunlight and shadow, and always give a front seat when things get intense. An *AVN* award-winning series, notably for #7 (1997), #8 (1997), and #12 (1999).

John Leslie's Voyeur's Favorites: Blowjobs and Anals

A compilation of his favorite blow job and anal sex scenes; won an *AVN* award in 1997.

Naughty Wives Club series

Sean Michaels, the leading African-American actor/director, gathers together a diverse selection of beautiful women for his excellent wall-to-wall series. While the filming style is choppy in select scenes, with a stylized feel that makes it seem like a few frames a second are missing, the excitement of the female performers shines through. You get the feeling that the women are in the films because they just like Michaels so much, and their happy, smiling sweaty faces are a testament to how much fun they're having. Diverse bodies and body sizes, occasional scenes with slow-hand lover Michaels, and several different film styles make this series interesting and refreshing.

DIRECTOR: Sean Michaels, series began in 2000.

NYC Underground series

Joe Gallant's blend of situationalist performance art and hot 'n nasty amateur New York women make his tapes unique in every way from the rest of the adult industry. Footage of lesbians acting out in front of riot police in New York are side by side with Gallant and a horny, shaved New York girl, another woman nervously laughing and giving herself public paint enemas on a dark street in New York, and more minimalistic but very real and very fevered sex. Some tapes contain extreme fetishes and sex acts; check the box cover for contents.

DIRECTOR: Joe Gallant, series began in 2001.

NOTE: S/M activities with sex.

Woman Penetrates Man

Natural Cast

Unsightly Boob Job

Well-Made Film

Real Female Orgasm

Real Female Masturbation series

Randy West directs this series of women masturbating for the camera, with a special focus on the women demonstrating exactly how they like to masturbate—for the camera, anyway. Scenes range from public masturbation and first-time toy experiments, to porn amateurs and female ejaculations. Authentic and enjoyable.

DIRECTOR: Randy West, series started in 1998.

Rocco's Animal Trainer series

Italian rough rider Rocco Siffredi operates gonzo-style, picking up lovely European women and having extremely athletic, rough sex. The theme is that the women are crazed sex animals who need hard sex, and there is liberal employment of whips and chains, rough anal sex, and Rocco's trademark wild-man enthusiasm and fetishistic glee for the women's asses and feet. Rocco's heavily-hung European sidekicks join in. Some feature first-time starlet debuts, and the action verges more toward the kinky than in most other all-sex tapes. Heavy focus on anal sex.

DIRECTOR: Rocco Siffredi, series began in 1999.

NOTE: Foreign release

Rocco's Reverse Gangbang 1 and 2

The reverse gang bang isn't what I'd hoped—a bunch of women pushing Rocco Siffredi around, demanding orgasms until they are through with his limp, lifeless body. No, instead it's Rocco's fantasy, a dozen women doing what he says and passively receiving his rimming, vaginal, and anal attentions. Other men join in, and female pleasure is definitely not the focus here, but lovers of group scenes will enjoy these raw European productions and Rocco's clear passion for his work. No safer sex, minimal production values, little editing, and after the reverse gang bangs there are more sex scenes so that you get your money's worth.

DIRECTOR: Rocco Siffredi

#1, 2001, 137 min.

#2, 2002, 125 min.

NOTE: Foreign release.

Dominant Women

Violet's Top Choice

Intense Chemistry

Extreme Sex Acts

Great for Newbies

Screaming Orgasms series

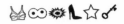

Wall-to-wall women, alone, in pairs, and threesomes, all doing one thing: masturbating themselves and each other to orgasm. Real orgasms. The women talk to the camera, sometimes emitting jaw-dropping dirty talk, then get off on fingers, vibrators, dildos (sometimes really big ones), and a Sybian sex machine, which is reminiscent of those coin-operated buckin' broncos found outside supermarkets in the 1960s—but with dildos in the right places. The production values are unpolished, but the performers steal the show with their mesmerizing orgasmic displays.

DIRECTOR: Various, series started in 2001.

Shane's World series

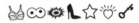

When women take the reins and make their own gonzo porn, you'd better look out—and grab the lube. Performer Shane started *Shane's World* by renting a motor home, gathering together her sexually aggressive starlet pals, and hitting the road for a little R and R, outdoor sports, and loads of indoor sports that included lots of T and A. From there, the adventures continued with the mobile home, on vacations to river hideaways, and everywhere else Shane's ever-changing ensemble cast of starlets wanted to get some action. The most notorious adventure: the 2002 *Campus Invasion* (#32), where Shane and the gang went to one of the top schools in the country to party and shoot porn, and wound up making headlines. The name of the game with Shane is nasty fun, with the women calling the shots and getting off, and performers who look like your everyday, average white college kids.

DIRECTOR: Shane, series started in 1996.

Shane's Pornological

This series is fantastic for so many reasons, and the really bad, tongue-in-cheek humor doesn't hurt—or help! The theme is that "life is an experiment," and the viewer is treated to many salacious experiments, such as a married couple having sex for Shane's camera, acrobatics, odd segments such as "when porn stars attack," and more hot sex than you can shake your stick at.

DIRECTOR: Shane

Woman Penetrates Man	Natural Cast	Unsightly Boob Job	Well-Made Film	Real Female Orgasm

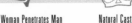

Joey Silvera's Rogue Adventures/Big Ass She Male series

Top-quality wall-to-wall "chicks with dicks" action, with great production values; transsexuals with generous butts, breasts, and dicks; and performers who are really having a good time. The combinations include solo masturbation, two tranny women together, male with tranny gal, two gals together, trannies with biological women, and group scenes.

DIRECTOR: Joey Silvera, series started in 1998.

Skin: Flesh series

Not quite wall-to-walls, but more like compilations of loosely themed vignettes, this European collection has nice production values, good-looking male and female performers, and at least a couple of especially arousing scenes on every tape. The Euro actors all look like attractive models. While the heat varies from scene to scene, some of the films excel—*Skin: Flesh #8* is particularly good, focusing on public encounters. Production quality is overall decent, though some are badly dubbed. The better ones aren't dubbed at all. These are a terrific choice for those looking for wall-to-wall couples' sex without typical porn actors, sets, or formulas.

DIRECTORS: Various (Eurotique Entertainment), started in 1995.

NOTE: Foreign release.

Strap-On Chicks series

The first installments of this female-penetrating male series featured performers who appeared to be amateurs, yet the recent videos have performers such as infamous starlet Belladonna (*Strap-On Chicks: Bella's Bitches*). The women often are extremely rough with the men, forcing them to suck their dildos and penetrating them with large strap-ons. Sometimes there are good scenes with chemistry and excitement, and the occasional "love sandwich" with a guy in the middle, but sometimes the scenes are lackluster and disappointing.

DIRECTOR: Various, series started in 1998.

| Dominant Women | Violet's Top Choice | Intense Chemistry | Extreme Sex Acts | Great for Newbies |

Video Virgins series

This series features young women having sex in front of the camera for the first time, though the women are usually already sex performers of some type. Still, the masturbation is real and the orgasms authentic, and it's enjoyable to see them tune out the presence of the camera so they can concentrate on coming. Some are shy, others demonstrative, and the combinations include masturbation, couplings with women and men, and oral and anal sex.

DIRECTOR: Various, series started in 1993, won an *AVN* award in 1994.

Randy West's Up N Cummers series

A former male performer, Randy West now spends his time behind a camera making gonzo porn, while often performing in his own videos. He finds beautiful women who aspire to be porn stars, interviews them so you get to know them, and films (and fucks) them live, unedited. He has an enjoyable style with the women, and you can expect something different on each tape, such as outdoor urination, or a scene (*sans* West) with a real-life couple. Most have never been in front of a camera before, though many are professional strippers.

DIRECTOR: Randy West, series started in 1993; won *AVN* awards in 1994, 1996, 2002.

Woman Penetrates Man

Natural Cast

Unsightly Boob Job

Well-Made Film

Real Female Orgasm

S/M Features

My husband and I were getting into S/M, so we went to our local video store to rent a bondage tape. It was okay, but there was no sex! I thought we were supposed to be renting porn…

S/M is a blanket term for sadomasochism; bondage and discipline (B/D); role-playing; and dominance and submission (D/S)—and nowhere is that term more of a blanket than in S/M videos. Such videos can cover all this ground and more within a single tape, giving the viewer a front-seat ride through whippings, spankings, and hot wax treatments; exquisite Japanese rope restraints that look like works of art; women dressed as nurses or cops doing unspeakable things; and men who will do anything to please their mistresses. You can see outrageous—and extremely expensive—rubber and leather outfits adorning stern and beautiful dominatrixes, or skintight latex wrapped around the curvy asses of doe-eyed submissives. Some of the most-skilled experts in S/M can be seen using the poise and techniques that make them so good at what they do, and in many how-to videos on the market pros like these show you how to try S/M at home, safely.

But much of what you'll find here is eye candy, gas for the flames of your own fantasies and scenarios. Need an idea for an evening of pleasurably torturing the one you love? Pick up an S/M how-to video, which mixes instruction with scenes designed to get your creative juices—and other juices—flowing. An S/M video can introduce a new idea into your relationship, perhaps opening up channels of communication that can take you closer to making your fantasies reality. Or perhaps you already enjoy S/M and just want some additional stimulation, or masturbatory material that speaks to your personal preferences. And maybe you simply think that women in fetish gear look hot—it's all here, in the world of S/M videos.

There are, however, a few things missing from S/M videos. For one, S/M videos suffer from many of the same complaints lodged against other porn features—technical problems like bad sound or lighting, ditzy porn stars with their "perfect" looks, and porn's minefield of unenthusiastic performers. A good S/M video (like the ones in the following review section) will have high production values *and* look like a visual feast for the eyes—because, among other things, S/M is so very visually arousing. A good video will show people who *look* like real people: sexy, sex-loving, and sexually alive in their everyday bodies (most S/M films include amateur performers). And a great S/M feature will have players who are skilled, and whose chemistry and lust for each other make you sit up in bed and cry, "yes, sir!" while your hand sneaks its way into your lap. But still, something's missing from all S/M films, something that makes each and every one of these films unrealistic: no S/M video features sex.

Why Don't They Show S/M with Sex?

But wait a minute—BDSM is a sexual practice, and porn is about sex, so why don't they show the two together? Those who practice and play with S/M know how hot and sexy these two great tastes are together, and renting an S/M tape with sexy players who do nothing more than spank each other in rubber outfits can be pretty disappointing. Unfortunately, in the eyes of the law, anything outside of vanilla sex is considered "edgy" content—even though many regular folks engage in these edgy sex games every day. The problem is, many lawmakers believe that S/M and sexual practices such as fisting are harmful—they simply don't understand what these practices really are. And contrary to what the lawmakers think, S/M *isn't* about abuse, degradation, or non-consensual violation, such as rape.

In reality, the sensual rituals and games that fall under the title "S/M" are for people who respect and trust one another. People who engage in S/M experience the thrill, rush, and arousal that come from an agreed-upon exchange of power. One lover holds down her sweetheart's hands while she administers loving spanks to his naughty, gleefully wriggling behind; a couple can dress in leather, lingerie, or uniforms and play erotic games of dominance and submission with sexual rewards; one partner can enjoy surrendering to the feeling of restraint and allow herself to be sensually whipped into erotic bliss that can only come from surrender, fantasy fulfillment, and intense physical stimulation. Her partner can tap into the forbidden erotic charge that comes from wielding absolute power over another's pleasure—and pain. Sex and S/M in combination can make for the most unforgettable, mind-blowing, pivotal, emotional, and even spiritual sexual experiences you can imagine.

In the United States, laws regarding sexually explicit material serve to keep pornographers and retailers on their toes, never knowing for what, or when, they might be prosecuted for offending "community standards." You see, the law in the U.S. states that something is considered "obscene," and therefore illegal to create or distribute, if a court somewhere says it is. You might hear people in and out of the adult industry say things like, "Showing urination is illegal," or "Showing S/M with sex is illegal," or "Portraying Joan Rivers as a fashion expert is illegal" (and if it isn't, it should be)—and all these cautious statements are incorrect. In fact, there's only a single test, which is when a court in any of the fifty states decides that a particular thing (tape, book, picture, washed-up comedienne, whatever) is, by the "standards of the community," obscene.

No one making S/M videos knows if what they are doing is illegal or not. That is, until they receive a sweet invitation called an "indictment" and attend a party just for them called a "trial," followed by a big hang-over called a "conviction." Then they've been (albeit arbitrarily) bad. This situation, reminiscent of organized crime tactics, is not an oversight; the U.S. Supreme Court is quite aware that the only way that retailers and pornographers can really be sure they won't be prosecuted for sell-ing "obscene" material is for them to avoid portraying activities that might possibly be interpreted as obscene—*anywhere*. So meanwhile, the courts seem smug and pleased with themselves, conservative politicians can trot out a pet cause when the polls are flagging, and the retailers and creators of the most widely recognized product in America (outside the 99-cent hamburger) sweat through every single business day—while the government never actually makes smut categorically illegal. Based on caution and court cases, adult retailers know that they cannot ship S/M and sex videos to Alabama, Indiana, Kentucky, Mississippi, Nevada, North Carolina, Tennessee, Texas, and Utah as well as the northern district of Florida.

The topic of obscenity is, put lightly, a slippery slope. If you're like me and you survived the National Endowment for the Arts debacle where performance artist Karen Finley faced off against ultraconservative Senator Jesse Helms's frightening stance on obscenity in art, then you're likely to be wary about the notion of others defining your individual standards of obscenity. Merriam-Webster's dictionary defines "obscene" as "1: disgusting to the senses: repulsive; 2A: abhorrent to morality or virtue; *specifically:* designed to incite to lust or depravity; B: containing or being language regarded as taboo in polite usage; C: repulsive by reason of crass disregard of moral or ethical principles (an *obscene* misuse of power); D: so excessive as to be offensive (*obscene* wealth, *obscene* waste)."

In a court case for obscenity, the accused is held to whatever the local community's standards are for obscenity, as determined by a jury. The real question is, whose morality or virtue is being offended here? A jury sitting there worrying about how much work they're missing while stuck in court? The many people who bought or rented the tape? And whose community standards come into question when you're talking about a consumer product? Attorney General John Ashcroft found the exposed breast of a statue in the halls of his own Justice Department to be obscene, and ordered it covered up. *I* find the one-million-dollar per episode salary for each cast member of *Friends* to be obscene (that was twenty-two episodes per season, folks). But an act of mutual sexual pleasure between adults? Please—spare me, *and* my tax dollars.

So legality and porn is a big crapshoot for retailers and pornographers. In many cases producers have decided to avoid material that could cause problems, though some are willing to take a chance and portray sexuality in a more diverse and realistic light, and ready to face the consequences. In my opinion, I say let the consumers decide—keep the courts out of it.

Two Favorite S/M Directors: Maria Beatty and Ernest Greene

Whatever directors' and producers' legal fears and challenges may be, the realm of the S/M film has fostered filmmaking styles that fly beyond the imagination of many makers of more-regular, prosaic, adult fare. S/M films transgress typical porn, go where glossy music videos dare not go, and leave you with images that will erotically haunt you for days afterward. Two directors thriving in the subgenre of S/M films and leaving indelible marks on our viewing consciousness with their films are Maria Beatty and Ernest Greene.

Maria Beatty

Our fascination for the fatal, deadly beauty inherent in some women has no outlet in mainstream pornography. All too often in explicit films we find that the portrayal of erotic feminine power is cheaply done, has no meaning to the woman play-acting dominance for clueless directors who just want to make a buck, and lacks any threat or danger through either intelligence or femininity. Seeking the untouchable woman who inflames the dark side of our sexuality within film-noir aesthetics, we're lucky to find the films of independent New York filmmaker Maria Beatty.

Her short films have been the delight of film festivals and a sexual accelerant for S/M aficionados worldwide. Fostered by subjects such as bondage, submission, the silent film era, fear of the unknown, and lesbian contact, Beatty has created a legacy of films that delight in the playful relationship between pain and desire. Her adult films are a breed apart—they're dark, eloquently lit, and shot on film, and they showcase real-life dominants and submissives. With her dramatic lighting, taste for heady feminine S/M themes, and penchant for using black-and-white stock, she has the gothic-erotic S/M market cornered. A lifestyle submissive herself, she often appears on the receiving side in her own films, displaying intimate knowledge in her cinematic storytelling of succumbing to sexually powerful women. Beatty takes the fetish film, the S/M film, and the lesbian vampire film to a higher plane using dramatic lighting, high production values, authentic performers, plus her tendency of using black-and-white film. Her films seem to dwell in the shadows not only visually, but also by playing on the themes of perversion and lust for erotic destruction at the hands of another woman. In essence, she whips up tasty morsels for indecent but smart appetites.

Ernest Greene

Inevitably, we traipse into the porn section at the video store looking for a hot S/M video and come home with a poorly shot, unconvincingly acted home movie with players dressed in awful outfits. What we really wanted was something glossy and sleek with scenarios like short stories, acted out by experienced professionals wearing real fetish gear, experiencing authentic pain, and showing genuine devotion to their obsession. In the films that come from the mind of wicked Southern California S/M director Ernest Greene, we find those things exactly—and a filmmaker who is willing to push the rules.

If you're looking for a great S/M director, you can't miss with Greene. He has lashed his way to the top of the heap in the realm of mainstream adult S/M videos with authentic performances from actors, cool plots that are not unlike scenarios from contemporary books, and an unflagging, unassailable wit in his own screen appearances. Plus, unlike the usual S/M porn crap, his dominatrixes are *real,* and it shows. Be aware that his casting pool of submissives is mostly artificially endowed porno actresses—albeit ones genuinely into S/M—but the viewer quickly forgets about this as the dommes solicit heart-stoppingly true submission from them.

Greene knows the truth about S/M—that it's a turn-on, that it's sexy, and that when it's done right it makes you want to fuck like bunnies—and regularly comments on the industry's unwillingness to mix sex and S/M. His films show us a director who knows a thing or two (or a thousand) about S/M, plus women who love their roles and really want to fuck each other and who exude genuine chemistry onscreen.

Seeing Ernest Greene on film (and you occasionally will in other people's films—his are mostly all female), you'll see a skilled dominant, a startlingly creative mind, and a hilarious, cynical sense of humor. He looks just like turn-of-the-century silent filmmaker Erich von Stroheim, who had a serious reputation for sin: films that portrayed excesses in spending, strange fetishes, dominance and submission, a reputation for using real alcohol during prohibition, and closed-set orgies. In Greene we find Stroheim reincarnated, set free to enjoy the exploration of unusual fetishes, elaborate costumes, and the talents of highly skilled lifestyle dominatrixes against the backdrop of L.A. gloss. Elegant canings, spirited ponygirls, electrical play, and psychological predicaments are common themes in his films. For a change, we see them done well.

In 1998 Greene made a few wonderful films with Mistress Midori. Caught somewhere between the direction of Greene and the quiet authority and grace of Midori, a group of L.A. porn actresses transcend their own boundaries—even prompting Greene to remark in surprise after the completion of the films. He has recently partnered up with Nina Hartley, in film and in real life, and they are making great films together.

Educational S/M Reviews

Fetish FAQ series
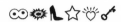

Dominant Ernest Greene teams up with well-known L.A. dominatrix Mistress Ilsa Strix to present this excellent series that imparts a wide array of knowledge on specific subjects. Each video begins with Greene and Strix on a couch discussing S/M, and while Strix wanders with dialogue, Greene dishes out info like a sushi chef at dinner hour. Then, with the premise of answering questions from fans via each dominant's website, viewers get a series of vignettes with professional players (and porn stars) who answer questions and solve dilemmas. Fun, engaging, arousing, and full of info, with both male and female dominants and submissives.

DIRECTORS: Greene and Strix

Fetish FAQ 1: Bondage How-To for Loving Couples, 2000, 70 min.
The first installment is high in chemistry and focuses on bondage, domination, and erotic torture for couples.

CAST: Alex Foxe, Chloe, David, Deva Station, Ernest Greene, Jack, Ilsa Strix, Randi Rage, Ryan Moore

Fetish FAQ 2: Breast and Nipple Play, 2000, 67 min.
Breast bondage, nipple torment, and all things boob are explored, including a great scene with Greene and Chloe solving the conundrum of breast play on women with small breasts.

CAST: Ernest Greene, Mistress Ilsa Strix, Chloe, Deva Station, Randi Rage, Alex Foxe, Ryan Moore, David, Jack

Fetish FAQ 3: Spanking, 2000, 71 min.
Naughty boys and girls beware: This is a complete primer on spanking. Men and women get paddled in this very arousing installment.

CAST: Ernest Greene, Mistress Ilsa Strix, Deva Station, Randi Rage, Alex Foxe, Chloe, Ryan Moore, David, Jack, Sydnee Steele

Fetish FAQ 4: Bondage, 2000, 65 min.
Ropes and restraints are demonstrated on some very wiggly submissives, and once they're tied up we learn how to torment captives to orgasm, using a variety of toys that include nipple pumps and vibrators. Great female orgasm scene.

CAST: Ernest Greene, Mistress Ilsa Strix, Deva Station, Randi Rage, Alex Foxe, Chloe, Ryan Moore, David, Jack

Woman Penetrates Man Natural Cast Unsightly Boob Job Well-Made Film Real Female Orgasm

Learning the Ropes series

Porn performer Ona Zee and her husband produced and directed this series of S/M how-tos that are cast with porn stars and shot with extremely low production values. These tapes cover much specific information (such as dealing with male submissives) that other tapes don't. The information is helpful as an add-on to S/M books and other videos, and though the performances are genuine, note that they are over ten years old (expect dated everything) and the quality is rough, rough, rough.

DIRECTOR: Ona and Frank Zee

NOTE: Independent filmmaker.

Learning the Ropes 1, 1992, 85 min.
Male submissive, spanking, restraints, foot worship.

Learning the Ropes 2, 1992, 79 min.
Male submissive, cock and ball bondage, whips, cross-dressing, dildos.

Learning the Ropes 3, 1992, 78 min.
Male submissive, advanced techniques.

Learning the Ropes 4, 1992, 68 min.
Female submissive, spanking, ropes, restraints.

Learning the Ropes 5, 1992, 79 min.
Female submissive, whips, feathers, canes.

The Pain Game

Highly regarded French BDSM educator Cleo DuBois tells you—and shows you—how to set up and negotiate a scene, then gets to work on a female and male submissive in two separate scenes. Her style is truly inspiring, as she's truly a loving dominant, and her instructions during the intense scenes are beyond what a book can tell you about S/M. The horny male sub is treated to genital clips and whips, and the female's back is decorated with piercing needles after a sound whipping. Not for beginners.

DIRECTOR: Cleo DuBois, 2000, 54 min.

CAST: Cleo Dubois, Creed, Brad Chapman

NOTE: Independent filmmaker.

| Dominant Women | Violet's Top Choice | Intense Chemistry | Extreme Sex Acts | Great for Newbies |

Tie Me Up!

Mistress Cleo DuBois gives indispensable guidance on making scenes sizzle and flow well from start to finish, while showing you exactly what she means in three scenes that drip with lust and chemistry between Cleo and her submissives. Talk about devotion! A scene in which she tops a male dominant is electric, and at the video's conclusion, Cleo shows you exactly how to tie those fancy knots.

DIRECTOR: Cleo DuBois, 2002, 52 min.

CAST: Jana, Jack, Alexis, Cleo DuBois

NOTE: Independent filmmaker.

Whipsmart

The elegant and beautiful San Francisco professional dominatrix Mistress Morgana hosts and gives hands-on instruction for couples who want to learn about S/M. It's an excellent primer for the beginner, has a terrific overview of what's included in BDSM practices, and clearly gives Morgana's definitions of terms and practices. It's well-shot and cast with very happy participants, including a lesbian and a male-female couple.

PRODUCTION HOUSE: Good Vibrations/Sexpositive Productions, 2001, 82 min.

CAST: Mistress Morgana, Butch, Vivian, Kanchan, Brain D, Buck Young, Lulu

NOTE: Independent filmmaker.

Woman Penetrates Man

Natural Cast

Unsightly Boob Job

Well-Made Film

Real Female Orgasm

Lesbian, All-Girl S/M Reviews

For more girl–girl sex mixed with light S/M and high fetish (plus the occasional man used a sex object), see Andrew Blake in Chapter 8, "All Sex, No Plot."

Bittersweet

This beautiful short is akin to the films you'd find in the independent section at your video store: lovingly made and poetically shot. Real lesbians who are clearly crazy about each other portray a dominatrix who comes home and relieves her slave's erotic tension. Play piercing and flogging are what's for dinner. Difficult, though not impossible, to find.

DIRECTOR: Alice B. Brave, 1993, 18 min.

CAST: N/A

NOTE: Independent filmmaker.

The Black Glove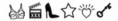

Like a black-and-white silent film, this stunning film is a heady mixture of shadow and gloss, and as far away from L.A. porn as you can get. The erotic tension is at an all-time high in this short tale about a young submissive (Maria Beatty) who will do anything to please her gorgeous mistress, played by Mistress Morgana. With a subtle, moody sound track, we watch spanking, foot worship, hot wax, and some of the most expressionistic devotion caught on film.

DIRECTOR: Maria Beatty, 1996, 30 min.

CAST: Maria Beatty, Mistress Morgana, Sabrina

NOTE: Music by John Zorn. Independent filmmaker.

Dark Paradise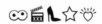

Shayla LaVeaux plays a fetish artist who draws her dream mistress, bringing Mistress Midori to life in exquisite scenes of Japanese rope bondage, canings, and over-the-top ponygirl service. The all-star cast is clearly eager to show their adoration to Midori.

DIRECTOR: Ernest Greene, 1999, 89 min.

CAST: Mistress Midori, Shayla Laveaux, Raylene, Roxanne Hall, Candy Roxx

Dominant Women

Violet's Top Choice

Intense Chemistry

Extreme Sex Acts

Great for Newbies

The Elegant Spanking

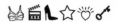

High art meets feminine D/S in this gorgeous black-and-white film, which through mesmerizing visual storytelling shows the punishment of a housemaid by her mistress. Haunting and arousing, in the mood of a Fritz Lang film, the scene includes submission, foot worship, urination, and yes, a very elegant spanking.

DIRECTOR: Maria Beatty, 1995, 30 min.

CAST: Maria Beatty, Rosemary DeLain

NOTE: Independent filmmaker. Music by John Zorn.

Ivy Manor series

This has to be one of the most elaborately costumed fetish and S/M series ever made, complete with full rubber deprivation suits, detailed pony gear, and outrageous rubber maid costumes. The tapes follow Jennifer, a journalist who talks her way into a strange academy for girls and winds up—to her pleasure—as a submissive to the mistress. But Jennifer is naughty, and when caught in Sapphic bliss with other rubber-festooned subs, she's punished to extremes. Her naughtiness gets her sent to other dommes, and that's the thread tying the tapes together. All that, plus a terrific cast that exudes genuine relationships. The series is ten tapes long; these are the first four.

PRODUCTION HOUSE: Gwenmedia

CAST: Isabella Sinclaire, Jewell Marceau, others

NOTE: Independent filmmaker.

Ivy Manor, the Beginning, 2000, 57 min.
Unbelievable maid service, douche, enemas, sensory deprivation.

Ivy Manor 2, Jennifer's Initiation, 2001, 60 min.
She's bound, humiliated, and caught in *flagrante* licking honey off a hot blonde, then more sensory deprivation.

Ivy Manor 3, Tropical Submission, 2002, 60 min.
Sent to learn new behaviors from other mistresses, she's tied to a stake, spanked, gets hot wax, and is trained to be a ponygirl. This tape features slower pacing and effective mood development, making the pony scene eerie.

Ivy Manor 4, Continuing Education, 2002, 60 min.
Jennifer is back at school for more punishment, including whipping, dunking, clothespins, and mummification.

| Woman Penetrates Man | Natural Cast | Unsightly Boob Job | Well-Made Film | Real Female Orgasm |

Ladies of the Night (Les Vampyres)

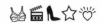

Les Vampyres begins showing a lost little schoolgirl (played by Beatty) who wanders frightened in an unfamiliar neighborhood. Next, she is whisked away to a richly appointed castle, awakening to find she is bound securely to a chair. From that point on, she becomes the plaything of two beautiful and squishy domme vampires, who torture her to their heart's content. The scenes are incredible, stunning in their approach as Beatty learns erotic body worship and is beaten, whipped, and caned before being subjected to penetration. In the finale, it's impossible to look away as plain-Jane Beatty is femmed-up, made over, and then made into one of *them*.

DIRECTOR: Maria Beatty, 2000, 32 min.

CAST: Mistress Dakota, Mistress Tchera, Bleu

NOTE: Independent filmmaker.

Prison World

It's an all-girl, all-porn-star B-movie about women in prison come to life—with explicit S/M and girl–girl sex. Great production values and terrific directing make this well-acted, very sexy film terrific, and the genuine lust and enthusiasm the performers have for the material is infectious. A female prison warden makes the most of her position in an all-woman prison that is actually an exclusive resort for wealthy submissive ladies.

DIRECTOR: Ernest Greene, 1994, 98 min.

CAST: Porche Lynn, Sarah Jane Hamilton, Misty Rain, Diva

NOTE: S/M activities with sex.

Dominant Women

Violet's Top Choice

Intense Chemistry

Extreme Sex Acts

Great for Newbies

Real Lesbians, Real Bondage series

Gritty and extremely rough, this series features scene after scene of real dykes and femmes going to town on each other, tanning each other's hides in a real San Francisco dungeon. The interactions are quite intense, and the range of styles from "andro" lesbians to pierced and tattooed baby dykes to butches and high femmes is true to real life, and not seen anywhere else in porn.

PRODUCTION HOUSE: Redboard Video

CAST: N/A

NOTE: S/M activities with sex, independant filmmaker.

Real Lesbians 1, 2002, 72 min.
Yee-ouch. Face-slapping, caning, dildo-fellatio, and femme subs brought to tears.

Real Lesbians 2, 2002, 60 min.
Leathersex is the dish of the day, with forced obedience to merciless femme mommies and butch daddies.

Real Lesbians 3, 2002, 62 min.
Dykes go at each other, with forced submission and dildo penetration, plus another scene with clothespins, humiliation, and tears.

Rope of the Rising Sun

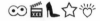

In beautiful Mistress Midori's first video appearance, she collaborates with Japan's incomparable master of rope bondage Takeshi Nagaike to bind and torment eager starlets. Ropes of every color, amazing works of human bondage art, and incredible suspended floggings are only parts of this well-shot, high-fetish epic.

DIRECTOR: Ernest Greene, 1997, 71 min.

CAST: Master Takeshi Nagaike, Mistress Midori, Jill Kelly, Randi Rage, Roxanne Hall

Woman Penetrates Man	Natural Cast	Unsightly Boob Job	Well-Made Film	Real Female Orgasm

S/M Reviews, General

For more S/M-themed features, lighter on the S/M but heavier on the sex, look in Chapter 7, "The Classics: Porn's Golden Age," for the titles *Emmanuelle* and *Story of O*.

Art of Bondage series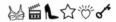

This series may be one of the most beautiful testaments to S/M on tape. These videos look like glossy fetish magazines come to life, with elaborate fetish wear and S/M gear. Real-life S/M players and couples (most are real-life lovers) engage in long scenes that are set to a low-key musical score. In addition to the burning chemistry between the players, breathtaking visuals abound, and the S/M covers a wide range of play styles, from spankings to electrical edge play. One of the rare series in which the box covers reflect the look and quality of the videos.

DIRECTOR: M. Zabel

CAST: Mistress Natasha, others

NOTE: Independent filmmaker.

Art of Bondage 1, Black-and-white, 1998, 60 min.
Two women delight in bondage and sensory play; a pair of anonymous male hands take a bound woman to the heights of breast torture; and a sexy, naughty woman is spanked and punished by her tall, stern boyfriend.

Art of Bondage 2, Color, 1998, 62 min.
A mistress spanks and whips two giggly, round-bottomed, misbehaving female submissives; a man enacts a medical scene with his submissive girlfriend that includes electrical play; the finale is a sensory deprivation, erotic suspension scene.

Art of Bondage 3, Color, 1998, 60 min.
Five scenes that include a female submissive bound to handicap rails in a bathroom, a male submissive tortured in suspension at the hands of the mistress in Vol. 2, a male dom roping up his female sub, a naughty gal having her bottom tenderized with paddles and floggers, and a final scene with elaborate sensory deprivation.

Art of Bondage 4 , Color, 1998, 60 min.
A busty submissive is restrained and menaced for her first time, a female submissive prepares her mistress's bedroom for erotic torture (which she certainly gets), and a male dom puts his female sub center stage for erotic punishment.

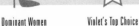

| Dominant Women | Violet's Top Choice | Intense Chemistry | Extreme Sex Acts | Great for Newbies |

Back Down

A lovely, young, and somewhat inexperienced dominatrix takes a variety of men to task in this gritty, bare-bones tape. Raven-haired Angelica spanks, paddles, humiliates, face-slaps, and is really, really mean to a variety of men, including Jamie Gillis, who, to the delight of this reviewer, gets the worst of her fury.

DIRECTOR: Duck Dumont, 1996, 60 min.

CAST: Angelica, Jamie Gillis, others

Bright Tails series

Although the budgets are low and the filming is amateur, the quality of Bob Bright's tapes are very high in terms of realism and performer enthusiasm. The well-groomed performers focus on each other and have a good-natured lust for S/M.

DIRECTOR: Bob Bright

CAST: N/A

NOTE: Independent filmmaker.

Bright Tails 2, 1993, 113 min.
Mistress Simone wakes up her bound slaves by dominating and punishing them in a variety of entertaining ways, including spanking, paddling, boot licking, nipple clamps, ice cubes, and various creative forms of bondage.

Bright Tails 3, 1993, 60 min.
A pretty gal with a round bottom suffers at the hand of her boyfriend until she's slick with arousal, then a couple consult a male dominant for erotic S/M instruction.

Bright Tails 4, 1994, 70 min.
Pairs of naughty female submissives get in lots of trouble with their male masters, and we get to see bondage, spanking, clamps, whips, and hot wax.

Bright Tails 5, 1994, 67 min.
An all-female tape, featuring Summer Cummings and Skye Blue, with lots of serious whipping and great chemistry.

Bright Tails 6, 1995, 60 min.
Stocks, ropes, paddles, and clamps feature in these three terrific female-sub, male-dom vignettes.

| Woman Penetrates Man | Natural Cast | Unsightly Boob Job | Well-Made Film | Real Female Orgasm |

Bright Tails 7, 1995, 56 min.

An expert dominatrix, a hot young submissive woman, and male submission make this tape sing.

Bright Tails 8, 1998, 62 min.

Corsets, tattooed gals, and an incredible female orgasm are the treats, along with a final scene of a bad boy being topped by two women.

Leda and the Swan...Nailed!

A contemporary setting for this Beatty film, this time a dungeon and an apartment, where Mistress Sonja Blaze discovers her submissive girlfriend spanking a boy-toy, sends the boy home, and sets in to punish the bad girl. Each toy the mistress uses causes the gorgeous submissive to have a flashback to a sticky scene with another juicy femme, a scene that includes extreme play with items such as knives and the barrel of a gun. Some pacing problems, but the scenes and atmosphere are eloquent.

DIRECTOR: Maria Beatty, 1999, 42 min.

CAST: Leda, Sonja Blaze, Tom Crimes, Ellen Benavides

NOTE: Independent filmmaker.

Painful Mistake

Minimal production values don't take away from the energy the amateur performers bring to this independent production. Young Gen-X types star in a lengthy encounter involving a male dominant topping a buxom, chunky and cute female submissive. Interestingly, the cast and crew met via the Internet before filming.

PRODUCTION COMPANY: Blowfish Productions, 1994, 55 min.

CAST: Lady Martha and Sir Stephen

NOTE: Independent filmmaker.

Dominant Women

Violet's Top Choice

Intense Chemistry

Extreme Sex Acts

Great for Newbies

Portrait of a Dominatrix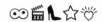

Elegant and always mesmerizing to watch, Mistress Midori stars in this faux-docudrama about her beginnings and evolution into the world-renowned domme she is today. A porn star cast performs the charming and all-male submissive scenes, which begin with a camera crew interviewing Midori as she recounts the highlights of her career. First comes Midori as a college girl who seduces, strips, and rides college professor John Decker like a pony. Then it's one scene after another with an enthusiastic and attractive cast who enjoy turning men into puppies, eliciting big boners with cock and ball torture, and spanking the hell out of every naughty boy in the film.

DIRECTOR: Ernest Greene, 1998, 60 min.

CAST: Mistress Midori, John Decker, Morgan Fairlane, Roxanne Hall, Anna Malle, Andy Parker, Hank Armstrong

Seduction: The Cruel Woman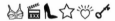

This amazingly beautiful, art-house German film never gets totally explicit in S/M or sex, but goes all the way with the erotic exchange of dominance and submission between the well-developed characters. A professional dominatrix humiliates male and female submissives for audiences that pay to watch, and when she breaks up with her lesbian lover a male submissive falls in love with her. This film is unique in many ways, but largely because it focuses on the psychology that is always at work behind BDSM relationships, even professional ones. Filmed in black-and-white with subtle blue sepia and some color.

DIRECTORS: Monika Treut, Elfi Mickesch; 1989, 84 min.

CAST: Mechtild Grossmann, Udo Kier, Sheila McLaughlin, Carola Regnier, Peter Weibel

NOTE: Foreign release.

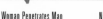

| Woman Penetrates Man | Natural Cast | Unsightly Boob Job | Well-Made Film | Real Female Orgasm |

Testify My Love

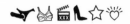

Elegantly filmed, with unrushed pacing and memorable scenes, this tense yet tender video explores male feminization and submission within the context of a love story. Young Tom wants to marry the woman of his dreams, and she is willing, but only if he will submit to all of her trials, including sissy maid service, sexual humiliation, blindfolded erotic torture, and losing his "virginity."

DIRECTOR: Maria Beatty, 1999, 42 min.

CAST: Marla Belt, Tom Crimes

NOTE: Independent filmmaker.

Thank You, Mistress

A young, modern Gen-X couple goes on a date to an erotic art photo show where they see pictures of S/M activities. The man comments that he'd like to try it someday, and she makes his fantasy come true, giving him to a cruel, sexy dominatrix for a session. Both beautiful, curvy gals take him to task, and then some, and the S/M-themed sex brings them closer together. Low budget, but great film style, plus a refreshing cast of trained actors with regular bodies but palpable passion.

DIRECTORS: Marianna Beck and Jack Hafferkamp, 2000, 35 min.

CAST: Mika, Poochie, Mistress Marilyn

NOTE: Independent filmmaker.

Dominant Women   Violet's Top Choice   Intense Chemistry   Extreme Sex Acts   Great for Newbies

10

Lesbian, All-Girl, Bisexual, and Gay Features

I'm a woman who likes her porn rough. Down and dirty, the filthier the better. I think all those people who soften porn for women are wrong—give me a dirty alley and hard anal sex any day!

When you first look at the title of this chapter, you might think that I've gotten my terms mixed up. Aren't lesbian and all-girl the same thing? It's important to distinguish between them and understand the definitions when you want to find porn that features women simply having sex together for fun, or women having sex together who are actually lesbians. The real world's terms, and the real world's sex practices, don't exactly jibe with how the adult industry labels these things—so knowing the difference will help you make the selection you want.

Every standard straight, or heterosexual, adult video contains an obligatory "girl–girl" scene—a scene in which two or more of the starlets have sex. When the makers of porn saw a potential gold mine in turning these obligatory scenes into full-length films, they created the "all-girl" market—and marketed the porn as "lesbian," though they certainly believed the likelihood of these films having an actual lesbian in them was slim to none. That's why real lesbians started making their own porn—because they like to watch porn, too, and they want to see lesbian sex that they would want to have, not films that were obviously packaged for men. All too often, girl-girl films deliver the producer's or the director's fantasy of lesbian sex—two girls bumpin' pussies—rather than authentic representations of real women having sex together. Interestingly, a significant number of women hired to portray the characters in these fantasies have girlfriends or have sex with women for pleasure as well as for pay.

Watching two women together is a powerful aphrodisiac, make no mistake. The all-girl videos show us an interesting and arousing side of female sexuality, and though many assume a male viewer, the women performers seem to relax more with each other. Some performers even regard bringing each other to orgasm as a game—and what a juicy game for two starlets to play! A good all-girl tape will have you absolutely glued to the screen, as you watch two women tell each other exactly how to make them both come—and then do it. If you're turned on by sex between women, it's as if a bolt of lightning hit your libido.

Real lesbian porn, by contrast, is where you'll see not only actual lesbians, but also a spectrum of female sexuality so diverse and powerful that you'll be blown away. And probably pretty turned on, too, because it's tough not to get aroused watching what you know is sex purely for the participants, rather than an act that by definition is staged. Porn made by and for lesbians is not for people who want to see bodies by Mattel, so consider yourself warned. In these videos you'll see all body shapes and sizes, hair or no hair, femmes and butches, women wearing strap-ons who exude masculinity, tattoos and piercings and virginal skin, and rarely a boob job. A totally different standard of beauty is at play here, and a different standard of sex, too. You're guaranteed an authentic female orgasm in every video, and furthermore these women have styles and methods of getting off that can't be matched by the adult industry with its formulas and scripts. Not to mention that most of the real lesbian films almost always feature real-life lovers.

Bisexuality, by definition, is sexual attraction to both men and women. So you'd think that "bisexual" films would show women with women, then men with men, and at some point everybody all together, like a sexually explicit version of *Bob & Carol & Ted & Alice*. But in porn, it's taken for granted that all the women have sex with each other for work, and so they're not considered "lesbian" or "bisexual." Hmmm. So it seems that bisexual films must be those that show two men having sex together but now and then going for a woman, or women. But the funny thing is, all bi films, with few exceptions, are made with gay male performers...so I guess the gay men are the bisexual ones, swingin' with women for pay. Confused yet?

Well, I promise you won't get too hung up on definitions when you see the unhinged lust that occurs in the boy–boy–girl three-way scenes —which are the raison d'etre of the bisexual genre. There's a reason that this type of porn is so in demand, and that's because when it's done right, it's red-hot. This is what the Roman orgies, and the ecstatic sexuality of truly decadent debauchery though history, were really about—men and women, crawling all over each other, not caring about who or what, with no hang-ups, just wanting to give and get as much pleasure as possible. Many people fantasize about two men screwing one woman (or more), and yet find it difficult to locate porn that is honest about the fact that all these people are willingly having sex with each other—and in the process deliciously, deliberately breaking all taboos. Yet it's entirely possible in the realm of bisexual porn.

Not all bisexual tapes are created equal, of course, not by a long shot. Straight porn is extremely homophobic. For straight porn usually features two men (or more) having sex with one woman, while desperately trying not to touch, or look at, or be aroused by each other. Conversely, bisexual films tend to be created with a certain distaste for the material—though it is a very popular, lucrative market—and as a result suffer in many ways. The filmmakers of bisexual material seem confused about who the audience is, and performances are generally robotic and lackluster owing to poor casting and lack of directorial enthusiasm. And all too many bisexual videos feature two men having sex with each other while desperately trying not to enjoy the female participants. However, some performers and directors do see the erotic potential in bisexual porn, and make incredible videos. You'll find a handpicked selection in this chapter, in addition to choice picks of real lesbian, all-girl, and gay male features.

Gay male videos make up a thriving industry unto itself. For people who get turned on by watching men have sex, gay videos are the place to see men genuinely enjoying their own (and each others' bodies), and having sex with pure, unfettered lust. The way the performers react to each other is unlike the exchanges you'll see in straight porn; in straight porn you seldom see eroticisim of the male body—men are not intentionally the primary sexual focus. For those who get turned on by male sexuality, this is a glaring omission. Gay porn can fill this void by portraying a man-to-man exchange that can be simultaneously hot, hard, unforgiving, and tender. Many men and women find it a complete turn-on to watch the beefcake, heavily hung, sexually supercharged porn studs give and get as much as they can take, and find there is a lot to be learned about male sexuality from watching gay porn—much more than what barely bubbles to the surface in straight porn. I can't count the number of times I've heard straight women exclaim over the gay video boxcovers how much sexier and more attractive the men in gay porn look as compared to straight male performers.

The gay porn industry is huge and wide-ranging, comparable in size to the straight porn industry. Many gay subgenres cater to dozens of individual preferences (with themes such as facial come shots, young meat, big balls, huge loads, beefcake, Latinos or Asians or African Americans, orgies, sports and jocks, bears and cubs), whole series devoted to fetishes, and a subgenre of plot-driven feature films, each with their own favorite directors. The budgets range from high to man-with-a-camera low, the themes from loving to unbelievably rough, and the men from smooth-young-boy-types to older, big, hairy bears. But usually what you'll see in today's gay porn is similar to straight porn's overly groomed cult of hairless youth in the form of muscle-bound beefcakes—a big departure from 1970s gay porn when, as in the "Golden Age Classics" of straight porn, everyone had lots of body hair or a mustache, and they didn't have waxed chests, hairless balls, gym-sculpted bodies, and perfect tan lines.

More is to be found in each of the genres listed below, and if you find what you like here, consult the "Resources" section, Chapter 14, to find even more. This may be a new frontier for your explorations, while for other readers, this is home.

Real Lesbian Videos

These videos feature real-life lesbians in realistic—as well as fantasy—settings.

Clips

Three short vignettes pack a lot of smut into a small amount of time, and feature real heat between the performers. Scarf bondage, an amazing female ejaculation, pussy spanking, and gender bending are a small sample of the highlights; the only regret is the poorly computer-digitized anal masturbation scene.

DIRECTORS: Nan Kinney and Debi Sundahl, 1988, 30 min.

CAST: Fanny Fatale, Coco Jo, Houlihan, Kenni Mann

NOTE: Independent filmmaker.

Full Load

Four scenes depict steamy scenarios that include exquisitely intense sex between lesbians, butch dykes, FTMs, and a whole host of queer women, and show us what's going down in the world of queer sex. Punk femme bitch tops make FTMs submit to their whims in a seedy abandoned bus scene; two butches in love have hard sex and wild orgasms; two queer women enjoy edge play that includes fire, asphyxiation, and giggles mixed with face-slaps; and an FTM and a femme in love have a wet quickie in a basement. Plenty of tattoos on the performers, plus lots of hot, grinding sex.

DIRECTOR: Barbara DeGenevieve, 2002, 90 min.

CAST: N/A

NOTE: Independent filmmaker.

Woman Penetrates Man

Natural Cast

Unsightly Boob Job

Well Made Film

Real Female Orgasm

Gallery Erotica

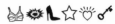

The viewer is taken on a tour of erotic lesbian photographs in a gallery, a clever plot device to make the photos come to life. The results are scene after scene of really searing sex with beautiful femme lesbians and attractive butches, shot beautifully and featuring incredible chemistry. In the vignettes, a buxom femme is seduced while watching lesbian porn; the gallery owner gets an hour of submission to her femme girlfriend; two French blondes in fetishwear are stranded roadside and must pee and have sex in public; and a butch gives a femme foot and shoe worship.

DIRECTORS: Alpha and Kurt Hardy, 2002, 60 min.

CAST: Angel, Cherry, Coyote, Dominique Devereaux, Kathryn MacGregor, Maîtresse Elise, Piper.

NOTE: Light S/M activities with sex. Independent filmmaker.

Hard Love and How to Fuck in High Heels

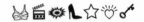

For those who want to see a well-shot, high-quality, real lesbian and butch dyke feature with lots of hot, intense sex, get this one right away. Two films in one, with the first vignette featuring a sexy butch and her gorgeous femme, and lots of sweaty, strap-on sex and incredible acting. The second is a faux-docudrama about femme Shar Rednour who gives instruction on strap-on fucking in high heels—a pale excuse to show her having incendiary sex with a curvaceous African-American woman and later topping the hell out of a submissive butch.

DIRECTORS: Shar Rednour and Jackie Strano, 2000, 96 min.

CAST: C. C. Belle, Tina D'Elia, Johnny Fremont, Jackie Strano, Josephine X, Simone, Chester Drawers, Shar Rednour, Jamie Ben-Azay, Nicole Katler, Edrie Schade, Veronica Savage, Arty Fischel, Stephani Rosenbaum

NOTE: Won an AVN award in 2000. Independent filmmaker.

Dominant Women   Violet's Top Choice   Intense Chemistry   Extreme Sex Acts   Great for Newbies

Home Cookin'

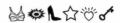

The all-femme cast is gorgeous and sincere, the acting terrific, and the sex super-fun and extremely arousing in this adorable story of love reclaimed. Rita runs a diner, and her BBQ is legendary, but when a curvy brunette with a hearty appetite comes in and sets her sights on Rita, it seems that the cook has taken love off the menu. But never fear, because soon her heart melts like butter and after some hot daydreams involving human feasts, the lovers unite.

DIRECTOR: Alpha, 2002, 48 min.

CAST: Maîtresse Elise, Katherine MacGregor, Roxanne

NOTE: Independent filmmaker.

Private Pleasures and Shadows

The mullets are breathtaking—and the orgasms are, too—in this video that delivers twice the action by framing a story within a story. A beautiful Asian lesbian is masturbating to lesbian porn, and the video reveals a magnetic butch/femme couple (a real-life couple) enjoying S/M and extreme acts of penetration, culminating in a love swing. Great care is taken in the production, and though the music isn't to everyone's taste, the passion of the performers is riveting.

PRODUCTION HOUSE: Fatale Video, 1985, 60 min.

CAST: Teri, Mariko, Caerage

NOTE: Independent filmmaker.

• •

Real Lesbian S/M

For real lesbian S/M films, check out:
> *Bittersweet*
> *The Black Glove*
> *Bright Tails #2*
> *The Elegant Spanking*
> *Ladies of the Night*
> *Real Lesbians, Real Bondage*
> *Seduction: The Cruel Woman*

For real lesbian educational films, check out:
> *Please Don't Stop*
> *She's Safe*

• •

Woman Penetrates Man

Natural Cast

Unsightly Boob Job

Well Made Film

Real Female Orgasm

SF Lesbians

Here is the real deal—all real dykes and lesbians, in a hard-core, wall-to-wall sex series. Butches, soft and hard; lesbians, lipstick and tomboy femme; bois and grrrls; and the whole hot spectrum of lesbian sexuality gets it on for the camera. Solos, couples, threesomes, shaving, piercing, strap-ons, pregnant lesbian Latinas gettin' off—even a dyke with a blow-up doll—in all kinds of scenarios and sex acts. Phew, how do you handle so much female sexual diversity? Grab a vibrator, that's how.

NOTE: Independent filmmaker.

Vol. 1, DIRECTOR: Michaela Reigus, 1992, 83 min.

Vol. 2, DIRECTOR: Michaela Reigus, 1992, 75 min.

Vol. 3, DIRECTOR: J. Jones, 1994, 80 min.

Vol. 4, DIRECTOR: J. Jones, 1994, 95 min.

Vol. 5, DIRECTOR: J. Jones, 1994, 85 min.

Vol. 6, DIRECTOR: J. Jones, 1994, 85 min.

Vol. 7, DIRECTOR: Amy Money, 1998, 85 min.

Vol. 8, DIRECTOR: Amy Money, 1998, 75 min.

Vol. 9, DIRECTOR: Cynthia Martin, 2002, 79 min.

Vol. 10, DIRECTOR: Cynthia Martin, 2002, 81 min.

Suburban Dykes

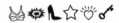

Even though this video has a cast of mostly porn stars, they got the sex and the butch–femme relationships right. Nina Hartley and Pepper play a suburban couple who try out a phone sex service for the first time, then go further by purchasing the services of an in-call dyke escort—oh, wonderful fantasy! Nasty sex, dirty talk, strap-ons, a hot three-way, and incredible orgasms make this woefully short video packed with action.

PRODUCTION HOUSE: Fatale Media, 1990, 30 min.

CAST: Nina Hartley, Sharon Mitchell, Pepper

NOTE: Independent filmmaker.

| Dominant Women | Violet's Top Choice | Intense Chemistry | Extreme Sex Acts | Great for Newbies |

SIR Productions

HOMEGROWN DYKE PORN with a professional edge is what you'll find in a SIR video, with real dykes and lesbians from San Francisco having sex the way it's really done—not at all like the girl–girl videos from straight production companies. With high production values, a wicked sense of humor, and a lust for butch dykes, femmes, and rough queer sex, the butch–femme team of this independent company are creating quality porn. But they don't only capture dykes on camera: In their runaway best-seller *Bend Over Boyfriend*, they show couples how to enjoy the fine art of female strap-on, male penetration; and in *Bend Over Boyfriend 2* they make the theme a wall-to-wall sexfest. With a viewership hungry to see themselves represented in porn, SIR has a bright future. Expect safer sex, sexy real-life amateur performers (with occasional porn star appearances, such as Chloe in *Bend Over Boyfriend 2*), lots of nonwhite cast members, excellent lighting and editing, and great, nonporn sound tracks.

Sugar High Glitter City

The directors of *Hard Love* made this gritty all-dyke fable about a city in the future where sugar is an illegal drug, and women will do anything to get it—including selling their bodies to mean dyke cops. There's a lot of rough play, tough talk, frenetic sex in dirty alleys, female ejaculations, and even some passionate sex between real-life partners. But it's all to get some sugar, baby. And those butches are way crooked cops.

DIRECTORS: Shar Rednour and Jackie Strano, 2001, 90 min.

CAST: Josephine X, Chester Drawers, Shar Rednour, Simone de la Getto, Hella Getto, Brooklyn Bloomberg, Aimee Pearl, Charlie Skye, Rocko Capital, Stark, Jackie Strano

NOTE: Independent filmmaker.

Woman Penetrates Man

Natural Cast

Unsightly Boob Job

Well Made Film

Real Female Orgasm

Voluptuous Vixens

Big, beautiful women pose, pout, and preen for the camera in a variety of retro-inspired settings to music, sort of like a low-budget Andrew Blake video—except the women have real, identifiable orgasms. Retro lingerie, cars, and haircuts, but modern sex toys, tattoos, and lesbian sex are all on this tape, a collection of scenes where the young women masturbate or bring each other off. The scenes are hit-or-miss, but when they hit, they hit hard, plus viewers can expect a diversity in ethnicity and body size not seen in a normal sexual context anywhere else in porn.

DIRECTORS: Sadie Foxe and Sadie Valentine, 2002, 85 min.

CAST: J. J. Belle, Cherise Soleil, Sadie Foxe, Olivia Luscious, Amy Money, Celestina Meow Meow

NOTE: Independent filmmaker.

All-Girl Videos

The subgenre known as "all-girl" or "girl–girl" videos features women-only sexfests, cast with porn starlets, made by mainstream porn filmmakers.

To see more girl–girl films that contain sex mixed with light S/M and high fetish (and an occasional man used as a sex object), check out the films of Andrew Blake cited in Chapter 8, "All Sex, No Plot."

Diva series

Master visual storyteller Ninn takes his penchant for stunning visuals and makes this already-intense collection of sex vignettes a feast for the eyes, put to music. The film styles vary to fit the scenes' mood, with clever use of color, lighting, and film stocks, and scenes are occasionally shot in back-and-white. Many feature big stars, and some of the scenes include fetish elements such as medical devices. The music in the series ranges from techno/ambient to hip-hop and even opera.

DIRECTOR: Michael Ninn

Diva 1 Caught in the Act, 1996, 102 min.

Ninn's first release focusing on sex between women is a series of fantasies in more than a dozen scenes, including sexual initiations and interrogation by dominatrixes.

CAST: Taren Steele, Juli Ashton, Jenna Fine, Kim Kataine, Vicca, Sindee Coxx, Sinammon, Monique DeMoon

Dominant Women	Violet's Top Choice	Intense Chemistry	Extreme Sex Acts	Great for Newbies

Diva 2 Deep in Glamor, 1997, 110 min.

Hot chemistry between performers and stunning costumes, with fantasies such as two brides and schoolgirls.

CAST: Cindy, Emanuelle, Felecia, Jill Kelly, Nathalie, Paisley Hunter, Ruby, Shayla LaVeaux, Stephanie Duvalle, Vicca

Diva 3 Pure Pink, 1997, 110 min.

Stylish "industrial" visuals and scenarios including apocalyptic outfits and settings such as freight elevators.

CAST: Nikita, Asia Carrera, Stacy Valentine, Roxanne Hall, Sunset Thomas, Paisley Hunter, Vanessa, Avalon, Malitia, Raven McCall, Solveig

Diva 4 Sexual Aria, 1997, 102 min.

Refined lifestyles are the theme, including an elegant feast for bedecked courtesans and a collared, leashed submissive worshipping a supermodel-type. Won an AVN award in 1997.

CAST: Nikita, Kia, Kim Kataine, Vicca, Tabitha Stevens, Asia Carrera, Jeanna Fine, Avalon, Stephani Swift, Morgan Fairlaine, J. R. Carrington

Femme 1 and 2

No plot here, just lovely Vivid starlets having plenty of hot sex together, in high-budget productions that feature lots of outdoor scenarios and plenty of authentic orgasms. The pacing is not rushed, plenty of dildos and anal toys are wielded, and some scenes have music. Femme 1 moves slowly, with scenes including bathtubs and role-play as pets. Femme 2 really sizzles with an all-water theme, which is terrific for the hot tub orgasms had by Chloe and friends, and a romantic outdoor bathtub scene, though it gets cheesy with a car-washing scene.

Femme 1

DIRECTOR: Jay Ashley, 1998, 81 min.

CAST: Candy Hill, Charlie, Felecia, Inari Vachs, Katie Gold, Montana Gunn, Monti, Randi Rage, Shelbee Myne, Teri Starr, Yvonne

Femme 2

DIRECTOR: Dyanna Lauren, 1998, 105 min.

CAST: Charlie, Chloe, Dee, Flower, Inari Vachs, India, Katie Gold, Kitty Monroe, Lisa Harper, Raylene

Woman Penetrates Man

Natural Cast

Unsightly Boob Job

Well Made Film

Real Female Orgasm

Four Finger Club series

This entire series is devoted to women who like it big, and who put on private unscripted performances for the camera in living rooms and bedrooms, in pairs and sometimes solo. Okay, they're not totally private shows, if you count the crew, but you know what I mean. Great production values and lighting, and the gals really enjoy putting on a show and being exhibitionists about their many authentic orgasms. And yes, four fingers is the standard here (no thumb or it's fisting—but who's counting?), though occasionally you'll see eight fingers (still no thumb), and lots of really big toys. Sometimes you'll see a big name here, just getting her start in adult.

DIRECTOR: Various, started in 1999.

NOTE: Occasional female ejaculation, won an AVN award in 1999.

The Good, the Bad, the Wicked

What's this? Lesbian porn western—a new cult genre perhaps? Anyway, extremely high production values make this parade of western clichés into pleasant viewing, especially for those who like stables, barns, dusty chaps, and strangers (Missy) who stroll into town to tell stories of sex-drenched days gone by. Unfortunately the music is not by Ennio Morricone, the sex is typical porn fare, the tan lines and racing-stripe pubic hair look pretty anachronistic, and some of the sex scenes fall flat.

DIRECTOR: Brad Armstrong, 1998, 85 min.

CAST: Missy, Charlie, Antonia, Stephanie Swift, Felecia, Shayla La Veaux, Nici Sterling, Ruby, Roxanne Hall, Shay Sweet, Dolly Golden, Kelsey Heart, Syren, Brooke, Mandi Frost, Randi Rage

Lick Me! series

This stellar all-girl, all-sex series doesn't boast big budgets or expert camera-work, but instead delivers a refreshingly racially diverse cast of women really enjoying the sex they're having and giving each other sweet seductions and mind-blowing orgasms. You'll see natural, amateur-type performers mixed with augmented pros, women of every color, settings that range from pools to offices, and hot sex with lots of passionate kissing. The accessories are toys; no rough stuff, bondage, or S/M themes.

DIRECTOR: Sean Michaels, started in 1999.

| Dominant Women | Violet's Top Choice | Intense Chemistry | Extreme Sex Acts | Great for Newbies |

No Man's Land series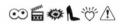

This series, which started in 1988, continues to today, with many spin-off series such as NML Interracial Edition Asian Edition, NML Behind the Scenes, and others ad nauseam. It was one of the first and is still the most archetypal of cookie-cutter girl–girl porn, though to its credit you can find favorite starlets having sex, yet it's largely hit-or-miss. Look for your favorite performers in newer editions, or find older editions for your favorite starlets in early performances, and you'll have a decent tape.

DIRECTOR: Various, series began in 1988.

Ooze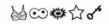

If you've seen the HBO series *Oz*, this spoof will make you giggle—until you watch the all-star cast get down to business in the "women's prison" scenarios, and you trade laughs for arousal. Newcomers to adult mix with the biggest stars from the last forty years to settle some scores, or at least dress and act like hardened female cons, talk rude and rough, and, er, give each other a good licking. Okay, it's not at all believable, but the sex is hot, raw, dirty, and hard.

DIRECTOR: Jim Steel, 2000, 90 min.

CAST: Tina Tyler, Jeanna Fine, Nina Hartley, Nikki Fairchild, Angelina De Carlo, Chloe, Rene Larue, Maya Divine, Chenine Blanc, Alexis Amore, Ava Vincent, Sharon Kane, Lauren Montgomery, Lola, Shayla La Veaux, Gloria Leonard

Shane's Slumber Party series

Female gonzo director Shane originally intended *Slumber Party* to be #6 in her *Shane's World* series, but it was so popular, she turned it into a series. Shane and her gal-pals have all-girl sex fests that feature lots of first-timers (who are usually strippers, so don't hope for too many all-natural amateurs). The sex is all over the map, ranging from light to rough (such as mild choking, but not S/M or bondage). They drink, wrestle, dare each other to try new things, play with vibrators and strap-ons, and even play Twister. And while some of the scenes seem to be for the camera, others are arousing, incredible, and authentic. The camera is handheld and the production values are minimal, but the scenes are well lit and clear. The cast resembles *Girls Gone Wild*, college girls, or women from MTV's *Spring Break*. A slice of whitebread America, the sexually adventurous girl next door.

DIRECTOR: Shane, series started in 1998

Woman Penetrates Man Natural Cast Unsightly Boob Job Well Made Film Real Female Orgasm

Sista series

If you like all-girl, all-sex series such as *Where the Boys Aren't* but would like to see an all African-American porn star cast, then this series is for you. Lots of big names here, and while you'll find disappointing scenes here and there, you can count on a few really hot scenes on each tape, with women who enjoy each other's bodies and love to have sex. Lots of toys and oral sex.

DIRECTOR: Various, series began in 1993.

Where the Boys Aren't series

When this famed series began, it was making a spoof on all-girl films. In the first installment (which won an AVN award), two directors want to shoot porn, and when the male performers are a no-show, they make a girl–girl flick instead, and the whole film is just fantastic. The series evolved and passed though many directors' hands, including skilled men such as Paul Thomas, Ernest Greene, and Brad Armstrong, with no consistency in plot. Each installment is high in production values and stars big names, some tapes have won awards, the sex seldom gets very rough (unless you consider strap-on sex rough), and the energy is high.

DIRECTOR: Various, started in 1990.

• • • • • • • • • • • • • • • • • • •

All-Girl S/M

For more S/M themed all-girl features check out:
Dark Paradise
Ivy Manor
Prison World
Rope of the Rising Sun

• • • • • • • • • • • • • • • • • • •

Wide Open Spaces

Very cute and sweet in every way, this all-girl video centers on adorable Kelly O'Dell, who moves to Montana to open a lesbian bar, get away from it all, and look for love. Each sex scene is tender and passionate, slowed down and genuine. No rough stuff, yet some of the best girl–girl chemistry in mainstream porn can be found on this tape.

DIRECTOR: Wesley Emerson, 1995, 100 min.

CAST: Kelly O'Dell, Nina Hartley, Misty Rain, Juli Ashton, Jeanna Fine, Sindee Coxx, Tina Tyler, Felecia

Dominant Women

Violet's Top Choice

Intense Chemistry

Extreme Sex Acts

Great for Newbies

Bisexual Videos

Bisexual videos are a popular genre where both men and women are objects of lust, heat, and sexual attention. Rather than a typical straight porn three-way where the men ignore each other's presence, the men in bisexual videos lavish equal attention on the women and each other, and the women fully enjoy the men's bodies, including anally penetrating their male partners. Fans of women donning strap-ons and plundering boys' backsides will find a gold mine of masturbation material here, while all viewers will see men and women getting it on without the usual formulas and homophobia found in straight sex cinema.

Biagra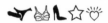

Don't let the low, low production values and the utterly ridiculous plot stop you from checking out this cute film. Two women experiment on their boyfriends—and every guy who crosses their radar (bi-dar?)—with some very interesting pills that make any man bisexual. Why? To have hot bi sex, of course, which they do. Tina Tyler has the hottest sex with her two gay neighbors, who obviously enjoy her affections—and her strap-on.

DIRECTOR: Karen Dior, 1998, 88 min.

CAST: Tina Tyler, Leo De Silven, Paul Carrigan, Dino Phillips, Alyssa Allure, Chris Danu, Michael D. Marco

Curious

The cute plot centers on two couples—lesbian and gay male—who become roommates, and realize that they're all a little curious about what it would be like to play for the other team. Although the "lesbian" couple isn't believable (and don't even watch the faked girl–girl scene), and a male ejaculation looks faked in the guy–guy kitchen scene, a hot three-way in an alley, a well-paced het scene, and a final group four-way all rate highly.

DIRECTOR: Anthony Rose, 1998, 85 min.

CAST: Tina Tyler, Candy Apples, Bunny Blue, Dino D'Marco, Herschel Savage

NOTE: Won two AVN awards in 1998.

Woman Penetrates Man	Natural Cast	Unsightly Boob Job	Well Made Film	Real Female Orgasm

Chi Chi LaRue

WITH HER MILE-HIGH HAIR, glitzy dresses and saucy attitude, drag queen director LaRue appears as though she'd be most at home in a John Waters film, or lounging poolside eating bonbons and sipping mimosas surrounded by beefy studs. Minnesota-born LaRue started directing, writing, and acting in gay porn in the late 1980s, and was quickly noticed for turning out films that had both style and substance. Her ability to coax genuine performances, convey character and motivation, and communicate her biting brand of tongue-in-cheek humor through story and action has only become more refined over the years. To this day she continues to make excellent gay and bisexual porn and win awards. Expect good-looking, enthused performers, excellent direction, and a polished film that might make you laugh hard—and come hard—at the same time.

Fly Bi Night

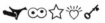

Sharon Kane wants to have a three-way with her boyfriend, so she watches him from a closet with another woman until she works up her courage…and the rest of this sex-packed video revolves around watching, and being watched. The finale comes when Kane blindfolds her boyfriend (straight porn star Julian, aka Jordan Rivers) and has another man fellate him, and when he sees what's going on, he first feigns dismay, then admits, "Sex is sex." Nice film, and several men with pierced tongues make effective use of the piercings with both men and women.

DIRECTOR: Chi Chi LaRue, 1997, 90 min

CAST: Jordan Rivers (Julian), T. J., Sharon Kane, Cory Summers, Sky Thompson

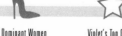

Dominant Women   Violet's Top Choice   Intense Chemistry   Extreme Sex Acts   Great for Newbies

The Hills Have Bi's

In this campy bi classic, hillbilly meets high class when horny housewife Sharon Kane's in-laws come for a visit. Lowbrow humor and hot sex, with a great seduction scene.

DIRECTOR: Josh Eliot, 1996, 85 min.

CAST: Sean Ryder, Lexi Eriksson, Jake Taylor, Drew Andrews, Taylor Dante, Paul Carrigan, Dylan James, Mason Walker, Alec Powers, Harley Peterson, and Sharon Kane; Harley Peterson, Chi Chi LaRue, and Moist Towelette in nonsex roles

Mass Appeal 1

The plot is thin—a wealthy bi couple cruise for off-duty soldiers in their limo to take home to their bi play-palace—but the quality of the film is exceptional. Great cinematography is courtesy of videographer Wash West, who was one of the finest gay filmmakers until his mainstream movie crossover, *The Fluffer*, and the great everything else is thanks to visually fueled direction by Michael Zen. To top it off, there's nary a lackluster scene, though not every scene is perfect.

DIRECTOR: Michael Zen, 1997, 85 min.

CAST: Ken Ryker, T. J. Hart, T. J. Cummings, Lauren Montgomery, Jon Eric

NOTE: DV, female spanking male, all-condom

Miss Kitty's Litter: Days Gone Bi

Yee-haw! This campy western features porn stars and gay beefcakes in the really Wild West, hammin' it up and havin' plenty of bi sex. Miss Kitty's bordello is the setting for all types of excuses for bi couplings, including a hilarious minister and his wife, Tina Tyler, who have a unique way of "laying on the hands." It's like a B-movie western on ecstasy and LSD, with plenty of blow jobs and anal sex. The orgiastic finale is pretty wild, too.

DIRECTOR: Chi Chi LaRue, 1999, 90 min.

CAST: Axel Garrett, John Hart, Alex Wilcox, Winston Love, Jack Reilly, Tina Tyler, Jose Davis, Mark Steel, Lauren Montgomery, Duncan Mills, Eric Jon, Haus Weston, Javier Duran

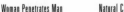				
Woman Penetrates Man	Natural Cast	Unsightly Boob Job	Well Made Film	Real Female Orgasm

Read Bi All
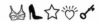

This is one of the more perfect bi films, in production quality, casting, chemistry, and hot, hot bisexual combinations. Scott Davis is a blond surfer-type who is working on a college paper about bisexuality. He decides to do research at the library, lorded over by the stern and gorgeous Tina Tyler. Davis falls asleep and dreams about a bisexual fantasyland with lots of intense sex. Later, the librarian invites him home for an interview with her, a practicing bisexual, and she has two men waiting for him when he arrives—making the final scene a scorching foursome, with all-natural Tyler being fingercuffed (see glossary) by the outrageously horny men. This film is exceptional in many ways, notably for a presentation of bisexuality with no hang-ups, a cast that can't get enough of each other, and portraying a woman who confesses to being bi.

DIRECTOR: Chi Chi LaRue, 1998, 90 min.

CAST: Cassandra Knight, Janis Jones, Tina Tyler, T. J. Hart, Joey Hart, J. J. Bond, Tom Adams, Anthony Stone, Rob Steele, Johnny Thrust, Scott Davis, Mitchell Stevens, Spike, Javier Duran

Remembering Times Gone Bi

With a nod to brat-pack films, a group of college friends get together for a weekend of reliving their memories, which all consist of sweaty, intense bi sex. The sex scenes are terrific overall, which won this video an award.

DIRECTOR: James C Stark, 1995, 111 min.

CAST: Sean Ryder, Lexi, Jake Taylor, Drew Andrews, Taylor Dante, Dylan James, Paul Carrigan, others

NOTE: Won several 1995 AVN awards.

Dominant Women

Violet's Top Choice

Intense Chemistry

Extreme Sex Acts

Great for Newbies

Revenge of the Bi Dolls

If you like the camp value of *Beneath the Valley of the Dolls* (Russ Meyer), then this hilarious send-up (loaded with fervent bi sex) has got your number. Bitchiness, jealousy, rivalry, and a drag queen/porn star mud wrestling scene are just a sample of this film's twisted, melodramatic highlights, and a cast that is really hot for bi sex doesn't hurt, either. They look like they had a lot of fun making this one.

DIRECTOR: Josh Eliot, 1992, 110 min.

CAST: Ty Fox, Tina Tyler, Sharon Kane, Gloria Leonard, Alec Powers, Vixxen, Vince Vouyer, Crystal Gold, Cort Stevens, Cutter West, Tony Idol, Dallas Taylor, Rob Baron, Chi Chi LaRue

NOTE: Won two AVN awards in 1994.

Slide Bi Me

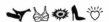

This independent film takes the art-house approach to bi films, combining a sur-real plot with a young, amateur, extremely enthusiastic cast to make a unique video. A company picnic goes awry and everyone has wild monkey sex with each other, sex that includes strap-ons, miscellaneous sex toys, and a slip 'n slide. The cast is all-natural, so folks who like skinny and shaved porn bodies should look elsewhere. The editing is roughshod and the music is awful, but it's a nice por-trayal of fun bi sex without the adult industry's usual baggage.

DIRECTOR: Felice Amador, 2001, 72 min.

CAST: Insertia Jules, Das Box, Kali Kream, Butch, Disel Velvet, Lisa Lixx, Candy, Sam Stern

NOTE: Less emphasis on male ejaculation; an independent film nominated for two GayVN awards. Independent filmmaker.

Woman Penetrates Man

Natural Cast

Unsightly Boob Job

Well Made Film

Real Female Orgasm

Gay Male Videos

Where's the beef? It's right here, in videos that give us hot, outrageously horny men who can't keep their hands—and everything else—off each other.

Against the Rules

This classic traverses a big taboo in its exploration of "sports stud being seduced by the coach" fantasy. And boy, is it hot! An academy cadet is discovered in the showers by his coach, who proceeds to seduce and totally ravage the very willing cadet—who, in turn, goes home to initiate his best buddy into the world of stiff dicks, hungry mouths, and eager asses. The boys like it so much, they decide that payback is in order and both pay a visit to the coach that results in a knee-buckling three-way.

DIRECTOR: Bill Clayton, 1980, 49 min.

CAST: Josh Kinkaid, Eric Nolte, Mac Turner

NOTE: No condoms, classic porn bodies

The Back Row

There are two versions of this classic film available, the condomless 1972 original and the 2001 scene-by-scene remake by top gay director Chi Chi LaRue. Both are fantastic, packed with hot sex and gripping lust. The recent version is shot-for-shot a tribute to the legendary original director Jerry Douglas. Typically, a Douglas film had a thoughtful plot, unheard-of budgets, amazingly strong, sexy actors, took up to two years to make, and cleaned up at gay awards ceremonies—and this video is a perfect example. Dark and low on dialogue, the film follows sexy blond Casey Donovan as he cruises for action in the back row of an adult theater, where he finds a handsome stud who then plays sexual cat-and-mouse with him all over Manhattan. A trip into a New York leather store, mild kink (such as dildos, candle wax and cock rings), icons such as sailors and construction workers, and frequent onscreen drug use represent the 1970s gay porn lifestyle. This film is a seamless construction of plot and sex, and while groundbreaking at the time, it is in many ways less explicit than today's gay porn.

Dominant Women	Violet's Top Choice	Intense Chemistry	Extreme Sex Acts	Great for Newbies

The Back Row, 1972 version

DIRECTOR: Jerry Douglas, 1972, 70 min.

CAST: Casey Donovan, George Payne, Robin Anderson, David Knox, Warren Carlton, Chris Villette, Arthur Graham, Robert Tristan

NOTE: S/M activities with sex. Music composed and conducted by William R. Cox. Independent filmmaker.

The Back Row, 2001 version

DIRECTOR: Chi Chi LaRue, 2001, 73 min.

CAST: Kyle Kennedy, Ryan Zane, Chad Hunt, Ethan Richards, Mark Slade, Dante Foxx, Rob Kirk, Danny Lopez, Thomas Bond, Tanner Reeves

Frisky Summer

These boys are barely legal and lovin' it! Young, just-18 men with uncut cocks frolic and fuck each other's brains out in beautiful, mostly outdoor European locations in this wall-to-wall feature. Each scene shows off their youthful bodies, and postadolescent sex drives, alternating tender and mildly rough sex.

DIRECTOR: George Duroy, 1995, 90 min.

CAST: Jon Daviddy, Johan Paulik, Milos Janek, Kristian Jensen, Daniel Valent, Tomas Belko, Dano Sulik, Gynt Klein, Alex Petersen, Filip Smirnov

NOTE: Foreign release.

Kansas City Trucking Co.

Director Joe Gage is the undisputed king of 1970s "rough trade" films, where truckers, construction workers, and all the classic working-man icons have tough (yet sensual), anonymous sex. This is the first installment in a series, where young hitchhikers are initiated in the ways of dominant truckers on the road, and in truck-stop bathrooms and backrooms.

DIRECTOR: Joe Gage, 1976, 70 min.

CAST: Richard Locke, Jack Wrangler, Steve Boyd, Kurt Williams, Duff Paxton, Skip Sheppard, Bud Jaspar, Dane Trennell

NOTE: No condoms, all natural bodies (no shaved genitals or other parts), and shot on film. If you like this one, see Gage's other terrific films, *El Paso Wrecking Corp.*, *LA Tool and Die*, *Handsome*, and his new films, *Tulsa County Line* and *Closed Set: The New Crew*. Cult classic.

Woman Penetrates Man   Natural Cast   Unsightly Boob Job   Well Made Film   Real Female Orgasm

Mardi Gras Cowboy

If you want to see gorgeous, contemporary Gen-X (nonbeefcake) guys having hot sex within a terrific plot, and throw a love story in to boot, then this is the film for you. Jim Buck is the (adorably) dorky hillbilly who thinks he can make it big servicin' the ladies in the big city as a stud-for-hire, but finds himself in one compromising situation after another—with men. It's hilarious watching Buck feign dismay and "do it for the money," utterly arousing to watch these sexy men have sex that's a cut above other gay vids in lust and chemistry. The love story thrown in for good measure is cute and believable. If they could all be like this....

DIRECTORS: Playa and Timco, 1996, 86 min.

CAST: Jim Buck, Vidkid Timo, Dan Kelly, Bod Simoneux, Gunner Johnson, Zod S., Sebastian X, Kevin K, Ken K, Jeffrey C, David J

NOTE: Independent filmmaker.

Matinee Idol

A great plot, excellent cinematography, and a well-acted script make this video a fun choice for an evening, and when you add the hot sex in every scene, you'd better make your evening a private one. Jeff Stryker plays a Hollywood star whose closeted gay life is about to come to the surface, and he's forced to decide whether he should deny or embrace his secret life. An excellent supporting cast with terrific chemistry round out this great flick.

DIRECTOR: Gino Colbert, 1995, 100 min.

CAST: Jeff Stryker, Ken Ryker, Christian Fox, Vince Rockland, Jake Andrews, Sean Diamond, Hank Hightower, Vic Hall, Chad Connors, Rob Cryston, Gio Romano, Jim Bentley

A Night at Halstead's

So sleazy and yet so hot, this roughly shot video takes the viewer on a trip to legendary gay male sex club Halstead's for a night of filling glory holes, jail scenes, and guys who want to show off how to make best use of a sex club—in every way possible. Leathermen and more, hurrah!

DIRECTOR: Fred Halstead, 1981, 75 min.

CAST: J. W. King, Fred Halstead, Greg Dale, Leo Thompson, Ben Barker, Robby Merton, Gary Sikes, R. J. Reynolds, Frank Romero, David Eagleton, Rick Lindsey, Mike Madera

 Dominant Women Violet's Top Choice Intense Chemistry Extreme Sex Acts Great for Newbies

Defiant Productions

IN STRAIGHT PORN, you can find amateur female masturbation videos populated by hotties who look like the cute girl at the local café. And you'll find plenty of tapes where these beginners "experiment" with their girlfriends—but where is the male equivalent? Where can you see everyday straight boys getting off? Defiant Productions has heard your pleas, and their several series of videos are here to help. With films that are shot quickly and have zero production values, they've "caught" dozens of straight skater boys jacking off (and trying a few new things with their friends) on video—and even if you don't think they're really straight, you won't care when you see the raw sexual authenticity in their scenes. Gen-X guys watch straight porn and jack off in their living rooms, skaters wank in public restrooms while looking at dirty magazines, and other young men get up to no good while their girlfriends are supposedly gone. Yes, they're the cute guys you see around the keg, on the half-pipe, and behind the record store counter—and they look even hotter when they masturbate. Favorite series include *Sportin' Wood, Curiosity* and *I Jacked Off Here*.

Night Walk: A Bedtime Story

In a stunning departure from his straight career, lush visual storyteller Michael Ninn teams up with gay director Gino Colbert to deliver a beautiful film that features sex with gargoyles, complete body shaving, flashbacks, flying divas, mansions, a chorus line, and more. In it, we follow a naïve young man as he is led through the underworld of male sexual desire. High production values surround the surreal characters and multitudes of hot and horny leathermen.

DIRECTOR: Michael Ninn, 1995, 96 min.

CAST: David Thompson, J. T. Sloan, Will Clark, Dino Dimarco, Chance Caldwell, Rob Cryston, Chad Conners, Ryan Block, Blue Blake, Paul Brazil, Cliff Parker, Mack Reynolds, John Romano, Rip Stone, Kevin Dean, Hank Hightower, Kurt Houston, Brian Maxx, Max Stone, Dane Tarson, Jon Dough, Jeanna Fine

Woman Penetrates Man

Natural Cast

Unsightly Boob Job

Well Made Film

Real Female Orgasm

Powertool

Jeff Stryker stars in this classic ode to jailhouse cock, and this film showcases Stryker's most famous assets—his big tool, and his skilled dirty talk. Rough sound doesn't detract from the many scenes of hot sex behind, through, and around bars, and pretty much every incarceration fantasy is given screen time. And, oh my, that soapy shower scene that results in a double anal penetration is an absolute blowout.

DIRECTOR: John Travis, 1986, 90 min.

CAST: Jeff Converse, John Davenport, Jeff Stryker, Michael Gere, Brian Estevez, Tony Marino, Gary Owen, Danny Russo, Tom Mitchell, Tony Bravo

NOTE: Won multiple AVN awards in 1986, no condoms.

Total Corruption 1 and 2 (set)

Cops (mmmm...uniforms!) and their homophobic hypocrisy are the target—and unending source material—for these humorous and hot videos that take the notion of "Vice Cop" all the way. In #1, a rookie gay cop can't believe what his fellow "straight" cops are doing to young men they bust on their beat—and gets a surprise when he takes the matter to his captain. But #2 makes the most of the hilarious camp possibilities within a homophobic cop context (not to mention jail scenarios) when a gay man is busted for cruising and brought in for a night in "the pokey," only to face off with the antigay sergeant.

DIRECTOR: Chi Chi LaRue, 1995, 180 min.

CAST: Greg Ross, Marco Rossi, Hank Hightower, Wes Daniels, Damian, Zak Spears, Scott Baldwin, Phil Bradley, Donnie Russo, Tom Katt, Scott Randsome, Hank Hightower, Blade Thompson, Tony Broco, Adam Wilde, Karl Bruno, Jordan Young, Hancock Blue, Chris Dano

Dominant Women

Violet's Top Choice

Intense Chemistry

Extreme Sex Acts

Great for Newbies

Educational Videos

I saw my first porn movie when I was 15. The star was John Holmes. He was enormous—and limp. For some time after that, I thought erections pointed down.

Sex education is not taught in our culture—at least adequately, and in a real-world context. Sure, many of us got a bit of birds-and-bees rhetoric in school, but the information had little to do with the questions we were beginning to face as adolescents, and was intended mostly as a stopgap measure by adults terrified of the consequences of not warning us about pregnancy and STDs. No one told us about exploring our—and each other's—bodies for pleasure, nor did they discuss issues we would face as adults navigating the seas of sex and relationships. Many people probably don't think that learning about sex, or how to have better sex, is something they can do as easily as renting a video. But as grownups, we have more options; we can weather through life and learn things by trial and error (pretty dangerous these days), we can read books about sex—or we can lie back and relax and watch sex education videos.

Sex education videos offer a wealth of information on sexual health and pleasure, in a variety of contexts, on a wide range of topics, and focusing on individual sexual preferences and orientations. You can learn female anatomy for pleasure—not reproduction—or how to give a man an erotic massage that will blow his mind. You can watch real-life couples demonstrate sexual positions that offer a variety of sexual benefits, learning and being titillated at the same time. Or you can get a hands-on tour of sex toys, or a lesson on making love to women given by porn stars. There are how-to tapes on oral sex, anal sex—you name it, and it's out there on tape. And if you haven't thought of it, some erstwhile sex educator is probably working on it right now.

Sexual how-to videos can be used in a variety of ways to enhance your sex life. Simply watching an erotic video can give you new ideas, strategies, or new knowledge that you can put into practice to improve your solo or partnered sex. Most of these videos contain explicit sex, and follow a formula of part education, part titillation, with demonstrations intended to turn on the viewer so he or she will want to try the techniques right away. Watching a sex ed video with your lover, as a lark, a serious learning experience, or even not seriously at all, can get you both turned on, give you fuel for new adventures, or introduce a new idea, such as trying oral or anal sex. Plus, watching a new technique and seeing how it's done is often easier and less anxiety-provoking than reading about it in a book, or having someone describe it to you.

Not all sex ed tapes are created equal. Many contain bits of inaccurate information, or make unfair judgments about other people's sexual practices. Because some education tapes are made by entrepreneurs, rather than trained sex educators, they can contain unsafe information as well. Buyer beware—but never fear: Many excellent videos are available, prepared by reputable educators and responsible production houses.

The quality of the information may be high, yet typically little money is put into sex ed tapes, so production values and budgets are usually (though not always) low. The result is many homemade-feeling tapes, all of them shot to video. They are usually taped in one setting, but some with higher budgets will be shot in different locations. Many of these tapes are labors of love, and the couples who do the explicit demonstrations are almost always real-life couples, whose chemistry is intense! Many from the bigger production houses will have a "talking head"—a sex educator/narrator who introduces the material and guides viewers through the scenes. The strange thing about sex ed videos is that they all feel really dated—even many made in the 1990s seem to have a 1980s feel. Consider yourself warned about big hair.

The following films are by no means all the educational videos available, but rather a sampling of the best tapes that contain information specific to sexual pleasure (for example, no massage videos fail to include genital massage techniques). They are grouped by sex act, not by sexual orientation, so you will find gay male videos in the anal sex section, and lesbian how-tos in the female sexuality section. How-to videos on S/M make up a vast subgenre, and you can find a selection of the highest quality S/M instructional videos in Chapter 9, "S/M Features."

Videos for Partnered Sex

Acupressure for Lovers

Acupressure is a healing art that stimulates nerve centers and releases tension by applying pressure to specific points, and you can bet that's really fun to try in a sexual context. This video shows you where to press and how long, to enhance specific sexual responses. Twelve pressure points are covered, and a 20-minute full-body erotic routine is demonstrated. No sex.

DIRECTOR: Michael Gach, 1997, 40 min.

CAST: N/A

NOTE: Independent filmmaker.

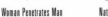

| Woman Penetrates Man | Natural Cast | Unsightly Boob Job | Well Made Film | Real Female Orgasm |

Ageless Desire: Great Sex for Couples Over 50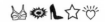

Juliet "Aunt Peg" Anderson presents and performs in this tape, which combines sex education about sex and aging with explicit sex between three older couples. The scenes run from simple erotic exchanges and sex to lightly kinky, S/M-themed encounters. The sex is explicit and the orgasms are focused, especially due to the couples' clear love and desire for each other.

DIRECTOR: Juliet Anderson, 2000, 55 min.

CAST: Juliet Anderson, others

NOTE: Independent filmmaker.

Better Sex for Black Couples 1 and 2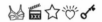

Black sex educators Shauna Croom and Herb Samuels explore cultural stereotypes, expectations, and myths about African-American sexuality and sex practices, then real-life, deeply loving couples explicitly enact seductions and sex techniques. Vol. 1 covers sexuality and seduction; Vol. 2 is packed with sex tips, positions, and fantasies.

PRODUCTION HOUSE: Sinclair Intimacy Institute, 1999, 60 min. (each volume)

CAST: Shauna Croom and Herb Samuels (nonsex), others

The Fist, the Whole Fist, and Nothing but the Fist

Porn starlet, notorious orgasm hound, and fist aficionado Chloe shares the joys of fisting with the world in this fun, information-packed, and arousing film. Shot in a let's-learn-as-we-go-along style, Chloe runs the show and first gives a group of a dozen women a lesson in fisting, then Chloe and another women show them how. Eventually everyone gets in on the fun, and at one point a dainty foot is substituted for a fist. This film is banned in the U.S., which seems weird when so many people enjoy fisting, and when it's perfectly okay to show eight fingers in a starlet, as long as they're not thumbs. See "Seymore Butts, aka Adam Glasser" in Chapter 8, for more information on fisting, and read the introduction to Chapter 9, "S/M Features," for the laws on fisting videos.

DIRECTOR: Patrick Collins, 2000, 78 min.

CAST: Chloe, Keisha, Felecia, Ruby, Charlene Aspen, others

| Dominant Women | Violet's Top Choice | Intense Chemistry | Extreme Sex Acts | Great for Newbies |

Nina Hartley's Guides to...Everything

THAT NINA HARTLEY may be one of the most beloved adult stars to ever grace the screen. With an infectious smile and a charming, effusive personality, she brings a sweetness and genuine presence to every scene she's in—and has the finest backside alive. While it's well known that she had an affair with her drama teacher while still in high school, few know that Hartley went on to college and graduated with a degree in nursing, magna cum laude.

Since then, Hartley has starred in over 650 films, including the notorious movies *Dirty Little Mind* and her first film *Educating Nina*. An outspoken critic of censorship, she tours the country giving lectures at colleges about her unique and quite strong views on sexuality, feminism, and pornography. In 1997, she shined in a small but pivotal role in the porn industry epic *Boogie Nights*. She has an entire line of exceptional sex education films, the *Nina Hartley's Guide* series.

Nina Hartley has made so many sex guides, it's a wonder she has time to make any porn. Her formula: Introduce the material, show needed diagrams or anatomy charts, then have her porn star pals strip down and try the sex act *du jour*, either all in the same room, or in scene-by-scene vignettes. It's a terrific way to present many of the subjects she discusses, in a loose format that is basically "sex tips from the pros." She begins with much-needed information (such as anatomy) to build a foundation for learning, and as she narrates through the sex, she presents more tidbits of information both from her and from the professional sex performers she's with. The only drawbacks are that with somewhat unscripted proceedings, the information can be haphazard, and the couples are really pros with no hang-ups, so you don't get a feel for what it'll be like for you to try it at home. And if you're not used to the comfort that porn stars have about open displays of sexuality, seeing Nina Hartley chatting with a woman while being penetrated or licked by her male partner can be a little odd. But there's nothing like her videos, since she's a former professional nurse she knows what she's talking about, and her works are chock full of solid information.

Woman Penetrates Man

Natural Cast

Unsightly Boob Job

Well Made Film

Real Female Orgasm

Joy of Erotic Massage

Step-by-step demonstrations with two extremely smitten couples show how to give incredible full-body and genital massages for both men and women. It's tough not to watch this video and be jealous about the massages the recipients are getting, and the narrator—though delivering priceless information—sounds like Barry White, which should get anyone's motor running. A fantastic tape with tons of information and a racially diverse cast.

PRODUCTION HOUSE: Sinclair Intimacy Institute, 2001, 60 min.

CAST: N/A

Nina Hartley's Guide to Seduction

Advanced foreplay, seductive communication, erotic dancing, and genital massage make up the highlights of the information here. Nina leads a group of women, porn stars and nonporn stars, though a guided erotic dance segment, then seduces one of the women, and we watch scenes where the women put their new knowledge to the test. Has a nicely diverse cast.

PRODUCTION HOUSE: Adam and Eve Productions, 1997, 120 min.

CAST: Nina Hartley, Midori, Missy, Aiko, Ty Law

Nina Hartley's Guide to Sex Toys

Hartley leads a small group of porn stars through a selection of toys and describes their uses, then the stars couple and use the toys as Hartley goes from couple to couple, discussing toys and techniques. The chemistry is hot, and the toy use is creative. However, Hartley enthuses about inserting a "vibrating egg" toy anally: Don't try this unsafe practice at home.

PRODUCTION HOUSE: Adam and Eve Productions, 2000, 87 min.

CAST: Nina Hartley, Dee, Inari Vachs, Marc Anthony, Ian Daniels, Angelica Sin

Dominant Women	Violet's Top Choice	Intense Chemistry	Extreme Sex Acts	Great for Newbies

Nina Hartley's Guide to Swinging

The methods and complexities of sharing and adding sex partners is the main topic of discussion, which Hartley speaks to with much personal experience. A vignette about novice swingers follows, and then a huge orgy.

PRODUCTION HOUSE: Adam and Eve Productions, 1996, 73 min.

CAST: Nina Hartley, Missy, Dallas, Shannon Rush, Bob Magnum, Luc Wylder, Alex Sanders

Ordinary Couples, Extraordinary Sex series

This fantastic and highly recommended series explores sex and intimacy in long-term relationships, discussing how to become closer and how to keep sex spicy over a lifetime through sex and communication techniques. Sex expert Dr. Sandra Scantling hosts, and real-life couples participate through discussion and display of intimacy and sex, though no genital close-ups.

PRODUCTION HOUSE: Sinclair Intimacy Institute, 1994, 60 min. each

CAST: Dr. Sandra Scantling (nonsex), others

Vol. 1 Discovering Extraordinary Sex
Strategies for improving communication and overcoming miscommunication, increasing trust and intimacy.

Vol. 2 Getting Creative with Sex
Creative erotic touch techniques, massage, sex games, and fantasy play.

Vol. 3 Keeping Sex Extraordinary
Advice and valuable information for long-term relationships.

Woman Penetrates Man

Natural Cast

Unsightly Boob Job

Well Made Film

Real Female Orgasm

The Sinclair Institute

SINCE 1991 THE SINCLAIR INTIMACY Institute has been working with sex educators and therapists to create a line of videos that help foster communication, teach sex techniques, and educate people about sex. Their videos cover everything from sex positions and specific techniques to erectile dysfunction and sex and aging. They use a combination of nonthreatening talking heads—well-coiffed therapists—and real couples explicitly demonstrating the subject at hand, to convey a clear understanding of the topics. The videos are often entertaining and full of great information, though the overall atmosphere feels oddly dated. This may be due in part to the fact that many of their films are from the 1990s, and the sets and digital cameras, coupled with the big hair, lingerie, and jewelry make quite a few of them feel like a daytime soap. But watching real couples with great chemistry and learning solid information can't be beat.

The Secrets of Self-Pleasuring and Mutual Masturbation

Masturbation is good for you and good for your partnered sex life, and this tape explains exactly why, as well as how to get the most from masturbation while in a long-term relationship. Male and female masturbation is explored with a narrator, and real couples demonstrate the techniques.

PRODUCTION HOUSE: Sinclair Intimacy Institute, 1999, 35 min.

CAST: N/A

Dominant Women

Violet's Top Choice

Intense Chemistry

Extreme Sex Acts

Great for Newbies

Sexual Ecstasy for Couples

Carol Queen is the effervescent tour guide for five young women on a journey into sexual exploration, who discuss their fantasies and how they have made them into reality—and how the viewer can, too. Fantasies include role-play, incorporating sex toys, power play, adding a lover, and more, and the discussion is spiced with explicit clips of the women putting their fantasies explicitly into play. Nicely shot, with very attractive couples.

PRODUCTION HOUSE: Libido Films, 1997, 62 min.

CAST: Dr. Carol Queen, others

NOTE: Independent filmmaker.

Sexual Healing: Finding Pleasure and Intimacy After Surviving Sexual Abuse

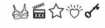

While not sexually explicit, this groundbreaking video is a must-see for anyone who survived or had a brush with sexual trauma in their lives—incest, rape, abuse, and more. Based on her workshops, somatic sessions, and her amazing book *The Survivor's Guide to Sex: How to Have an Empowered Sex Life After Childhood Sexual Abuse*, somatic practitioner Staci Haines steers this docudrama of examples taken from sessions of real-life men and women who have begun the journey of sexual healing. What sets this remarkable video apart—besides the unbelievable acting and life-changing information—is that its focus on healing revolves around creating a happy and healthy sex life as part of the healing process. We start out meeting six men and women in Haines's workshops and somatic sessions, and follow each as they learn to cope with reactions to sex such as fight, flight, freezing, and disassociation—and heal. Each situation is presented in a "not a perfect case scenario" context, making the outcomes realistic and authentic, and Haines includes many somatic exercises throughout the video for survivors to try at home—and tells what to do when the exercises don't work. The range of topics is astounding, including erectile difficulties, substance use, no interest in sex, when healing happens at different rates in relationships, and advice for partners of survivors of abuse.

DIRECTOR: Shar Rednour, SIR Video, 2003, 90 min.

CAST: Staci Haines, Howard Squires, Tina D'Elia, Melinda Wells, Christina Vickory, Maria Stanford, Kathe Izzo

NOTE: Independent filmmaker.

Woman Penetrates Man

Natural Cast

Unsightly Boob Job

Well Made Film

Real Female Orgasm

Sexuality Reborn

This amazing tape is the only tape of its kind, thoughtfully, tastefully, and intelligently providing a guide to exploring sex for men and women with spinal cord injuries. Four real-life couples share their experiences surrounding sexuality and injury, including dating, afterward lovingly demonstrating positions and tips for spontaneity. The strong focus on communication is invaluable information for everyone.

PRODUCTION HOUSE: Kessler Medical Rehabilitation Research and Education Corporation, 1993, 48 min.

CAST: N/A

NOTE: Independent filmmaker.

Talk to Me Baby: A Lover's Guide to Dirty Talk and Role Play

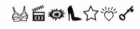

SIR Video's femme fatale Shar Rednour hosts a collection of rip-roaring, explicit, dirty-talk scenes that range from the sweet to the very kinky. She introduces the topic with her hip brand of wit and sass, then leads the viewer through becoming comfortable with hot talk and fantasy discussion with lovers, all punctuated by racy example scenarios that illustrate each point. Lesbian and het couples—mostly real-life couples—show a diverse range of fantasies, from a couple in bed dreaming of a rough biker scenario to a butch/femme couple playing "delivery man." Although it's technically an educational video, this tape packs in the wall-to-wall sex, with chemistry between the couples absolutely off the scale, a range of diverse bodies, and plenty of authentic female orgasms. The hilarious bloopers at the end are icing on the cake.

DIRECTORS: Jackie Strano and Shar Rednour, SIR Video, 2003, 60 min.

CAST: Shar Rednour, Sofia Carpaccio, Jack Manx, Jackie Strano, Tina D'Elia, Amy Pearl, Charlie Skye, Diesel Velvet, Butch, Chester Drawers, Simone de la Getto, Josephine X, Mistress Olive, Scott Blue

NOTE: Independent filmmaker.

Dominant Women   Violet's Top Choice   Intense Chemistry   Extreme Sex Acts   Great for Newbies

Tantric Guide to Better Sex

Tantra is an Eastern sexual practice that combines positions, breathing, timing, and mind–body awareness to heighten pleasure and prolong sex. This excellent tape is a great place to start, providing an expert discussion, feedback from couples who successfully use Tantra, and then explicit demonstrations of Tantric techniques. It's not for folks who want to fast-forward to the action; instead it's a thoughtful and carefully paced primer on unrushed sex.

PRODUCTION HOUSE: Sinclair Intimacy Institute, 1977, 60 min.

CAST: N/A

Guides to Sex Positions

The Complete Guide to Sexual Positions

With a little narration and explicit demonstrations by very happy, nineties-looking, real-life couples, this tape contains a hundred different sex positions in one hour. Wow! The emphasis is on one partner taking charge, and several of the positions afford G-spot stimulation. No genital close-ups or orgasms.

PRODUCTION HOUSE: Sinclair Intimacy Institute, 1995, 60 min.

CAST: N/A

Creative Positions for Lovers: Beyond the Bedroom

A diverse cast of real-life couples and narration by sex educators takes viewers through a whole lot of sex positions. See how adjusting an angle slightly can make a difference in comfort and pleasure, and view a host of positions for oral sex. Explicit, yet with no close-ups or orgasms; narrated by Bernie Zilbergeld, Ph.D.; Marty Klein, Ph.D.; and Linda Banner, M.S.

PRODUCTION HOUSE: Ultimate, 2000, 60 min.

CAST: Bernie Zilbergeld, Marty Klein, and Linda Banner (all nonsex), others

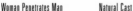

Woman Penetrates Man   Natural Cast   Unsightly Boob Job   Well Made Film   Real Female Orgasm

The Guide to Advanced Sexual Positions

With little time and a lot of chemistry, two real-life couples discuss and enact a terrific variety of sex positions.

PRODUCTION HOUSE: Sinclair Intimacy Institute, 1995, 27 min.

CAST: N/A

Oral Sex Guides

Better Oral Sex Techniques

Real-life couples explicitly demonstrate fellatio and cunnilingus, with narration by sex therapists Diane Wiley and Dr. Marty Klein. The video covers erogenous zones, positions, and pressure, and though I wish they'd show me how, they discuss but don't demonstrate deep-throat fellatio and 69. Sigh. Again, a good place for beginners to find info that helps them feel knowledgeable and comfortable.

PRODUCTION HOUSE: Pacific Media Entertainment, 1997, 60 min.

CAST: N/A

Complete Guide to Oral Lovemaking

This tape contains fifty-one oral sex techniques, explicitly demonstrated by non-porn couples. The look and feel of the video, hairstyles, lingerie, and jewelry is very dated, though the techniques are solid. The music and numbering of techniques is distracting at best, and the voiceovers explaining the techniques are unintentionally humorous. Good for beginners.

PRODUCTION HOUSE: Pacific Media Entertainment, 1997, 60 min.

CAST: N/A

Dominant Women   Violet's Top Choice   Intense Chemistry   Extreme Sex Acts   Great for Newbies

Nina Hartley's Guide to Fellatio, Cunnilingus, Oral Sex, Advanced Guide to Oral Sex

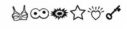

1994 was a very oral year for Nina Hartley. Adored by her fans, Hartley decided to give back what she was getting, and made four tapes that show her (and her porn star pals) dishing tips and demonstrating their tried-and-true oral sex techniques. In Fellatio and Cunnilingus, Hartley puts forth her knowledge from nursing and gives viewers a tour of male and female genital anatomy, then everyone gets down to business in group scenes, while she narrates and talks to performers during the action. Oral Sex combines the two and features more sex than instruction, though she gives tips and pointers throughout. Advanced adds onto tips from the first tapes, with genital massage techniques, a two-woman blow job, and an orally focused group scene at the end.

DIRECTOR: Nina Hartley

Fellatio, 1994, 45 min.
CAST: Nina Hartley, Alex Sanders, others

Cunnilingus, 1994, 45 min.
CAST: Nina Hartley, Angela Faith, Moose, Mike Horner

Oral Sex, 1994, 90 min.
CAST: Nina Hartley, Alex Sanders, Angela Faith, Moose and David, others

Advanced Guide to Oral Sex, 1994, 45 min.
CAST: Nina Hartley, Mandi Frost, Malitia, Tony Tedeschi, others

Woman Penetrates Man

Natural Cast

Unsightly Boob Job

Well Made Film

Real Female Orgasm

Anal Sex Guides

Bend Over Boyfriend

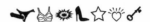

After watching the sales of dildos and harnesses to heterosexual couples continue to rise over the years, sex educators Shar Rednour, Jackie Strano, and Carol Queen felt it was high time to make a how-to video, and the result has been a best-seller ever since. As a cute film-within-a-film, two couples rent a how-to video about strap-on sex (featuring Queen and her real-life lover, Robert Lawrence) and when they watch it, they get inspired to try it themselves. The sex info is necessary, accurate, and on-target, and the couples shine with genuine lust.

DIRECTORS: Shar Rednour and Jackie Strano, Fatale Video, 1998, 60 min.

CAST: Dr. Carol Queen, Laura Goodhue, Cupcake Jones, Robert Morgan, Greg Heiman, Troy, Miss Behavin'

Note: Independent filmmaker.

Nina Hartley's Guide to Anal Sex

Hartley begins with the foundation of anal sex: anatomy and physiology. Then it's on to the porn stars to perform anal sex while she and the couple discuss (during sex) do's, don'ts, and tips to make anal sex for women easy, pleasurable, and exciting. This tape only focuses on anal penetration for women. Watching porn stars honestly engage in anal sex, with all the relaxation, arousal, and preparation necessary, provides excellent data for the novice and experienced alike.

DIRECTOR: Nina Hartley, 1995, 60 min.

CAST: Sinammon, Nina Hartley, Hank Armstrong, John Decker

| Dominant Women | Violet's Top Choice | Intense Chemistry | Extreme Sex Acts | Great for Newbies |

The Ultimate Guide to Anal Sex for Women 1 and 2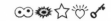

Anal sex guru Tristan Taormino hosts these educational/gonzo style all-sex tapes, and gives us excellent information about safe and fun anal penetration, with explicit demos by porn stars that go all the way. Tape 1 has Taormino dishing out tips and important information spliced with great sex scenes, including then-real-life couple Jazmine and Nacho Vidal, with an all-girl, all-booty orgy at the end. Tape 2 offers more sex than tips, as Taormino goes through each scene Nina Hartley style, talking to the stars about what they like anally while they get down to business. Shot by booty cam expert John Stagliano, the film has high production values and expertly lingering scenes, yet the tape falters when products are plugged repeatedly. But, for a tape that combines hot porn star sex, more sex acts than the main focus of the tape (including girl–girl scenes), and solid information, it's a rare and valuable thing.

Tape 1

DIRECTOR: John Stagliano 1999, 238 min.

CAST: Tristan Taormino, Nina Hartley, Chloe, Inari Vachs, Ruby, Sydnee Steele, Chandler, Jewel Valmont, Ernest Greene (nonsex), John "Buttman" Stagliano (nonsex), Tony Tedeschi, Nacho Vidal, Kyle Stone

NOTE: Won an AVN award in 1999.

Tape 2

DIRECTORS: Ernest Greene, John Stagliano, and Tristan Taormino, 2001, 135 min.

CAST: Bridgette Kerkove, Jewel D'Nyle, Jewel Marcel, Ava Vincent, Kate Frost, Lola, Tristan Taormino, Ernest Greene (nonsex), Joel Lawrence, Mickey G, Mr. Marcus

Uranus: Self Anal Massage for Men

This gay-male, spiritually-focused video by Joseph Kramer shows in loving detail men giving their posteriors the attention they deserve. Kramer blends Tantra and massage techniques, including healthy prostate massage, and the men practice relaxation and breath meditation as they explore anal penetration with the aid of vibrators and dildos. The video offers a New Age angle on opening up this often untapped pleasure zone.

PRODUCTION HOUSE: EROSpirit Research Institute, 1996, 40 min.

CAST: N/A

NOTE: Independent filmmaker.

Woman Penetrates Man

Natural Cast

Unsightly Boob Job

Well Made Film

Real Female Orgasm

Videos on Female Sexuality

Becoming Orgasmic

This explicit (though not sexually graphic) video is a step-by-step guide for preorgasmic women, or for women who have difficulty achieving orgasm. Although it takes its title from the excellent Betty Dodson book and follows the book's techniques, Dodson herself is not in the video. Female anatomy, touching for pleasure, and self-exploration are the main focuses, with a few suggestions for talking to your partner about sex. Narrated by sex therapist Joseph LoPiccolo.

PRODUCTION HOUSE: Sinclair Intimacy Institute, 1993, 83 min.

CAST: Joseph LoPiccolo, others

The Best of Vulva Massage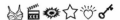

This collection of scenes from eight fantastic videos consists of the most comprehensive single video available on female genital massage, and is loaded with all kinds of practical—and pleasurable—information on stimulating a woman with your hands. From Tantra to postporn modernism, this video shows a variety of perspectives on female sexuality, and the knowledge combines with the visuals to give a thorough education. Clips from Betty Dodson's *Celebrating Orgasm*, Annie Sprinkle's *Sluts and Goddesses*, and Deborah Sundahl's *Tantric Journey to Female Orgasm* are just a few of the highlights. The DVD layers the information in an unbelievable amount of options: Multiple commentaries on each track by a number of respected and accredited sex educators take the understanding even further. It's possible to spend not just hours learning from the DVD, but possibly days or even weeks, not to mention the interviews with the many teachers. It's a refreshing and groundbreaking step for sex ed—rather than a talking head and some "action," we get scenes that shape our education with the many different perspectives of a diverse body of educators. Impressive!

DIRECTOR: EROSpirit Research Institute, Joseph Kramer, 2002

CAST: Annie Sprinkle, Betty Dodson, Julia Anderson, Jwala, Kenneth Ray Stubbs, Joseph Kramer, Deborah Anapol, Suzie Heumann, Jack Painter, Deborah Sundahl, Victor Gold, more uncredited

NOTE: Independent filmmaker.

| Dominant Women | Violet's Top Choice | Intense Chemistry | Extreme Sex Acts | Great for Newbies |

Carol Queen's Great Vibrations

Dr. Carol Queen is the resident sexologist at women-owned adult store Good Vibrations, and in this video she gives the viewer a very explicit tour through the full selection of vibrators the store carries (circa 1998). She explains each toy, how it works, and the pros and cons, and tries each one out, finishing with a G-spot ejaculation finale. She covers battery and electric vibes, clitoral stimulation, anal and vaginal penetration, vibes for men and women, and vibe care and cleaning. This is definitely the most complete video on the subject, though now a bit dated, and Queen delivers essential information for anyone interested in using vibrators.

PRODUCTION HOUSE: Fatale Video, 1998, 60 min.

CAST: Dr. Carol Queen

NOTE: Independent filmmaker.

Celebrating Orgasm

Women's sex therapist Betty Dodson does one-on-one counseling sessions with women, but they're not like any other—they're all specific to the women's orgasm issues, and include explicit advice. On this tape, five women allow their sessions to be taped, and Dodson counsels women whose needs range from wanting to change their masturbation style to a woman who has difficulty having an orgasm, period. Her advice is priceless, and watching the women try it on the spot (so to speak) gives revealing insights into the process and mechanics of female orgasm.

PRODUCTION HOUSE: Pacific Media Entertainment, 1996, 60 min.

CAST: Betty Dodson, others

NOTE: Independent filmmaker.

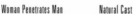

Woman Penetrates Man   Natural Cast   Unsightly Boob Job   Well Made Film   Real Female Orgasm

Expand Her Orgasm...Tonight!
A Pleasurable Program for Partners

Although the title makes an obnoxious promise, this video in fact demonstrates a creative assortment of female genital massage techniques that are geared toward orgasm. The very loving real-life couple have a deep connection that is arousing to watch, and the variety of techniques is unlike that in any other video, though the context of the information is near that of a well-produced home video. Explicit demonstration with female orgasms, and no male sex play.

PRODUCTION HOUSE: Pacific Media Entertainment, 1998, 60 min.

CAST: N/A

Fire in the Valley: An Intimate Guide
to Female Genital Massage

Sex guru, bubbly pleasure enthusiast, and former porn performer Annie Sprinkle teams up with Joseph Kramer to produce this fantastic guide to female genital massage. The techniques were developed at their New School of Erotic Touch over a six-year period, and cover both partner and solo genital massage. It's explicit, and though the strokes and rubs have New Age names that some might find goofy, the techniques are stellar and are demonstrated with refreshingly diverse women, including a lesbian couple and a man and his pregnant wife.

PRODUCTION HOUSE: EROSpirit Research Institute, 1999, 60 min.

CAST: Annie Sprinkle, others

NOTE: Independent filmmaker.

The Guide to G-Spots and Multiple Orgasms

Sinclair Intimacy Institute sex educators discuss and narrate G-spot anatomy and techniques, while a series of real-life couples explicitly demonstrate G-spot stimulation and orgasm through a variety of techniques, including manual and sex toy stimulation. Also includes information on male multiple orgasms.

PRODUCTION HOUSE: Sinclair Intimacy Institute, 1999, 60 min.

CAST: N/A

| Dominant Women | Violet's Top Choice | Intense Chemistry | Extreme Sex Acts | Great for Newbies |

How to Female Ejaculate

Porn performer Fanny Fatale hosts this extensive—and very graphic—guide to understanding and achieving female ejaculation. The women, many of them sex educators, discuss genital anatomy using charts and maps, then take a look at the real thing when Fatale uses a clear plastic speculum to open her vaginal canal. After they're done teaching viewers anatomy on the live model, the women talk about their ejaculation techniques—and then put them on display as they masturbate to ejaculation, all in the same room, and more than once.

PRODUCTION HOUSE: Fatale Media, 1992, 47 min.

CAST: Fanny Fatale, Baja, Shannon Bell, Carol Queen

NOTE: Independent filmmaker.

Incredible G-Spot

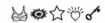

Laura Corn, author of sex tips books for couples, hosts and narrates this couples-focused how-to video on G-spot exploration. She employs the use of (now dated) computer graphics to illustrate anatomy points, and uses real-life couples who have tried her program and who discuss and demonstrate how well the techniques worked for them. Corn is like a G-spot cheerleader, though she covers all the essentials, and the couples honestly relate their adventures. The demonstrations are explicit with no genital close-ups.

PRODUCTION HOUSE: Park Avenue Publishers, 1995, 60 min.

CAST: Laura Corn, others

Nina Hartley's Guide to Making Love to Women

Hartley starts out with babe-a-licious Tina Tyler on the bed, talking about how to approach women seductively and sexually, with additional info from Tyler. A male audience is assumed, though there is a girl–girl scene, followed by a very cute heterosexual first-date sketch.

PRODUCTION HOUSE: Adam and Eve Productions, 2000, 140 min.

CAST: Nina Hartley, Tina Tyler, Jewel Valmont, Ian Daniels

| Woman Penetrates Man | Natural Cast | Unsightly Boob Job | Well Made Film | Real Female Orgasm |

Sexpositive Productions

WOMEN-OWNED SEX TOY STORE Good Vibrations has a video production arm, which makes a variety of education tapes (in addition to a couple of wall-to-walls). They use different directors and writers with each production, so quality varies widely and can be either rough and difficult to watch or excellent, with fantastic editing, great information, and sexy performers. They feature viewpoints not represented in mainstream porn, such as dyke safe-sex how-tos, or they take a topic such as learning S/M and give a fantastic introduction unique to people who love and practice the BDSM arts.

Please Don't Stop: Lesbian Tips on Givin' It and Gettin' It

Although made with minimal production values and edited possibly with a machete, this is one of the only tapes you can find that features a nonwhite cast of real lesbians discussing safer sex and sex toys, interspersed with scenes of the couples (and one sizzling solo) having sweaty, orgasmic—and gushing—sex. It is the first lesbian how-to sex tape made by and for lesbians of color. Diverse body sizes and age groups, and nice chemistry, provide a refreshing respite from porn standards, and the informal discussions on toys and lesbian sexuality provide a good overview—a great place to start. Music, with few genital close-ups.

PRODUCTION HOUSE: Good Vibrations/Sexpositive Productions, 2001, 74 min.

CAST: N/A

NOTE: Independent filmmaker.

Dominant Women

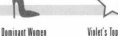
Violet's Top Choice

Intense Chemistry

Extreme Sex Acts

Great for Newbies

Secrets of Female Sexual Ecstasy

Charles and Carolyn Muir teach Tantric sex workshops, and in this video they host, narrate, and demonstrate a blend of Tantric and western techniques geared primarily toward female G-spot stimulation, though they include male ejaculatory control as well. This New Age film explores and demonstrates in great depth various Tantric sex techniques, and though it is explicit and shows real-life couples trying the techniques, it does not contain genital close-ups. The representation of body sizes and shapes is diverse, the couples are all heterosexual, the presentation feels slightly dated, and the focus throughout is on a New Age, or spiritual, perspective (for example, the G-spot is called the "sacred spot").

DIRECTORS: Carolyn Muir and Charles Muir, 1995, 80 min.

CAST: Carolyn Muir, Charles Muir, others

NOTE: Independent filmmaker.

Annie Sprinkle

WITH HER CUTE PIXIE FACE and sparkling brown eyes, this extra buxom brunette has single-handedly brought an awareness of sex and spirituality to both the adult industry and the general public, through her endless, sex-positive activism. Sprinkle's adult career began when she was a ticket-seller for an adult theater at the ripe age of 18. She soon found the industry to be a place where she could comfortably explore every type of sexuality she could dream up. She starred in many popular adult films, and many fringe epics that included all types of fetish sex.

Sprinkle graduated from the School of Visual Arts in New York City with a bachelor's degree in fine arts and graduated from the Institute for Human Sexuality with a Ph.D. in human sexuality. She's been in more than 200 films; worked as a prostitute for twenty years; lectures on sex, sex work, and pornography at colleges and universities across the U.S.; and has a one-woman show (and video) about her life and sexual awakening in the porn industry, *Annie Sprinkle's Herstory of Porn*. See great scenes of her in action in *Deep Inside Annie Sprinkle* and *Centerfold Fever*. Find out more about this amazing, multifaceted woman at her website, www.anniesprinkle.org.

 Woman Penetrates Man
 Natural Cast
 Unsightly Boob Job
 Well Made Film
 Real Female Orgasm

Selfloving: Portrait of a Women's Sexuality Seminar

For over a decade, sex therapist Betty Dodson taught workshops for women that explored female anatomy and sexual response in a group atmosphere, culminating in masturbation sessions that focused on learning and improving techniques. In this video, an entire workshop consents to allowing themselves to be filmed, and the result is an amazing document of these women's eye-opening explorations of their own—and each other's—bodies. The ten diverse women, whose ages range from 28 to 60, provide invaluable insights into female sexuality. This is an amazing video that offers a lot of information, both practical and priceless.

PRODUCTION HOUSE: Pacific Media Entertainment, 1991, 60 min.

CAST: Betty Dodson, others

NOTE: Independent filmmaker.

She's Safe

The Frameline Arts Foundation compiled this group of sizzling clips from lesbian-made, lesbian safer-sex how-to videos from the U.S. and England. The segments provide an excellent source for information on lesbian safer sex in a humorous and erotic context, as the scenes are all infused with a sense of humor and real-life lesbian lust. Includes scenes from *Well Sexy Women* and an appearance by Annie Sprinkle.

COMPILED BY: Frameline Arts Foundation, 1993, 65 min.

CAST: Annie Sprinkle, others

NOTE: Independent filmmaker.

Sluts and Goddesses Video Workshop

With wit and infectious humor, Annie Sprinkle shows that any woman can be a sex goddess, "in 101 easy steps." What actually happens here is that a fantastically diverse group of women get a sexuality makeover, starting with makeup and fashion tips, then end up stripping, doing pubic hair coiffures, finding their G-spots, and learning Kegel exercises. There's even a female ejaculation scene and one of Sprinkle's famous five-minute-long orgasms.

DIRECTORS: Maria Beatty and Annie Sprinkle, 1992, 52 min.

CAST: Annie Sprinkle, others

NOTE: Independent filmmaker.

Dominant Women	Violet's Top Choice	Intense Chemistry	Extreme Sex Acts	Great for Newbies

Viva la Vulva: Women's Sex Organs Revealed

Betty Dodson gathers ten women, ranging from 25 to 68, who discuss how they've come to feel about their vulvas. As if at a slumber party, the women primp their vulvas and put them on display as objets d'art, with Dodson showing each of them off, as Gothic, Art Deco, and more, and offering many tidbits of information about sexual pleasure and response.

DIRECTOR: Betty Dodson, 1999, 51 min.

CAST: Betty Dodson, others

NOTE: Independent filmmaker.

Well Sexy Women

Six British lesbians have a round-table discussion about woman-to-woman safer sex. We see demonstrations of safer sex in a series of romantic and arousing vignettes. A nice presentation of facts, as the women share information, rather than adopt the usual sex education video instruction format.

DIRECTOR: The Unconscious Collective, 1993, 55 min.

CAST: N/A

NOTE: Independent filmmaker.

Videos on Male Sexuality

Evolutionary Masturbation: An Intimate Guide to the Male Orgasm

Male masturbation is examined and oodles of techniques are demonstrated from a spiritual, healing perspective. Men show twenty masturbation techniques, including breathing exercises, use of toys, reflexology, "sex magic," and techniques to help prolong and deepen orgasm. Many demonstrations feature scenarios of ecstatic self-love, including semen tasting, and the three ejaculation scenes at the end are tastefully filmed.

PRODUCTION HOUSE: EROSpirit Research Institute, 1996, 45 min.

CAST: N/A

NOTE: Independent filmmaker.

Woman Penetrates Man

Natural Cast

Unsightly Boob Job

Well Made Film

Real Female Orgasm

Fire on the Mountain: An Intimate Guide to Male Genital Massage

Okay, this film, available on both video and DVD, is fantastic, but while the focus on gay male spirituality is refreshing and intent on healing, the music and New Age phrasing of the material verges on camp. But don't despair—Joseph Kramer demonstrates terrific male genital massage techniques developed over ten years at the Body Electric Massage School, which he founded. Possibly the most complete guide to male genital massage techniques ever made, the tape covers every arousing stroke form start to finish, explicitly demonstrated by men who love and adore each other's bodies. The original version, released in 1993, was 45 minutes long; the newer VHS version is 90 minutes long, and the DVD boasts an incredible three hours of instruction in male genital massage.

PRODUCTION HOUSE: EROSpirit Research Institute, 2003, 90 min.

CAST: Joseph Kramer (nonsex), others

NOTE: Won an AVN award in 1993. Independent filmmaker.

Nina Hartley's Guide to Making Love to Men

Hartley starts out on a bed with beefcake porn stud Herschel Savage, giving tips on seducing men, addressing myths about male sexuality, and teasing the hell out of her man. Then it's on to romancing and sexing guys, with lots of sex tips dished out by Hartley and displayed by her cohorts.

PRODUCTION HOUSE: Adam and Eve Productions, 1999, 100 min.

CAST: Nina Hartley, Dayton Rains, Kaylynn, Justine Romee, Ian Daniels, Herschel Savage

Solo Male Ecstasy

Lengthy masturbation scenes, which feature interesting strokes and use of toys, all the way to ejaculation are mixed with light narration and interviews. The awful music sounds like a video game soundtrack, but if you turn it down you have a hot tape of guys jacking off—or a nice visual instruction on male masturbation.

PRODUCTION HOUSE: Pacific Media Entertainment, 1996, 60 min.

CAST: N/A

Dominant Women

Violet's Top Choice

Intense Chemistry

Extreme Sex Acts

Great for Newbies

12

Safer Sex in Porn

I used to rent a lot of group scene porn, but I'm watching it less and less because I just can't believe that what the actresses are doing is safe. I mean, how are they not catching anything?

The notion of safer sex in porn seems oxymoronic for some, and simply moronic for others. Many who are familiar with STDs and viruses such as HIV are well aware of the transmission risks, and see the practices in porn—even with the minimal condom use—as a crazy and possibly deadly game of Russian Roulette. Meanwhile, those viewers who don't know anything about what's at risk when imitating the practices onscreen are unwittingly learning how to spread disease, unaware of the risks—and precautions—that performers take as well as ignorant of the realities of the business.

Porn is great for exploring our own sexual fantasies and getting off, but it is certainly not a source of accurate sex information. Choosing to watch porn that depicts unsafe sexual practices—and being turned on by it—does not make you an accessory to unsafe behavior. You are watching fantasy enactment to get off, period. Enjoying films featuring unprotected sex is nothing to feel guilty about, and remember that you will never really know the circumstances surrounding what you're watching, or the relationships of the performers (or their health status, for that matter). So enjoy your porn, and live your fantasies to their fullest, but be smart when you want to make your own fantasies come true.

Sex Practices in Porn

Safer sex in porn is hotly debated by everyone involved. Some companies and directors have a condom-only policy, many leave it up to the individual performers, and some are firmly against condom use because it "interferes" with their portrayal of sexual fantasy—even though in today's culture, where safer sex is a reality that many of us have grown up with, condoms and latex gear have become eroticized by a significant percentage of the populace. On the other hand, the erotic fantasy of unprotected sex is equally powerful for those of us who came of sexual age in the era of deadly, sexually transmitted viruses.

Be aware that condom use doesn't prevent every infection, disease, and virus. And in the manner in which condoms are generally used (with the exception of smarties like Ed Powers of *Dirty Debutantes* fame) there is much room for error. In fact, when condoms are only used for penetration and when the man ejaculates on a woman's external genitalia, the participants have pretty much undermined the use of a condom altogether.

In porn sex you'll also see many activities that are unsafe, even dangerous. Consider the fetish for ass-to-mouth contact, using everything from penises and fingers to sex toys—entire series are even devoted to the practice. Ass-to-mouth contact puts the recipient at great risk for

contracting hepatitis A, which can be treated but not cured; the penetrator is at no risk in this situation. Hepatitis A comes from getting fecal
matter in the mouth, and many starlets reduce their chances by taking
multiple enemas before anal sex scenes, though this is far from a foolproof measure. Anal-to-vaginal penetration is another sex act commonly
seen in today's porn, which by bringing bacteria from the anus to the
vagina can cause a bacterial infection, called bacterial vaginosis. Again,
enemas are used beforehand, but this practice too is not a reliable
safeguard.

While these warnings and descriptions of unsafe practices are sober-
ing, the adult industry has its own self-regulating testing policies in place
for performers. AIM Healthcare, for one, is a nonprofit agency offering
HIV and STD testing, gynecological services and treatment, counseling of
many types, and informational services for sex workers and the general
public—though it specializes in serving the porn community. AIM
Healthcare serves more than 400 clients a month and is making plans to
expand. Since its inception, the organization has successfully lowered
the spread of HIV in the porn industry, and has certainly increased
awareness among performers. By industry standards, an adult entertainment worker must be tested for HIV/AIDS every thirty days, and
standardizing tests for other STDs are on the horizon as much of the
industry now supports mandatory testing for chlamydia and gonorrhea.
Most—though not all—producers and directors refuse to hire an actor if
he or she lacks AIM's written record of an HIV test less than one month
old. However, since the industry is self-regulating in all aspects of testing
and condom use, safer-sex risk assessment ultimately falls into the hands
of the performers themselves: their precautions, their lives. Read more
about AIM, its testing procedures, and the history surrounding AIM's
inception in Chapter 5, "Common Concerns About Porn."

Sometimes, at home or onscreen, anal penetration occurs with
objects or sex toys that do not have a flared end, or a means to prevent
them from being accidentally pulled into the anal canal and lower colon.
The sphincter muscle is involuntary, meaning that it contracts and pushes
and pulls things in and out of its own volition, without your control.

• •

"Safer Sex"

YOU MIGHT BE WONDERING why I'm using the term *safer* instead of *safe* to indicate the practice of using barriers and proper lubrication to prevent injury and the spread of disease. That's because using barriers (such as condoms), even in our personal lives outside of porn, is not 100 percent foolproof in protecting each participant from contracting an STD or virus from sexual contact. Many factors are involved in every sexual encounter, and each party takes and assesses risks in each situation, "risks" including judgment calls made in the heat of the moment—or when the cameras are rolling. So safer indicates merely that safe-sex gear is safer than nothing.

• •

Having a sex toy with a flared end prevents the toy from being pulled inside, where it will become irretrievable. Once something goes in and doesn't come out, you must go to a doctor so you do not die from having something lodged in your colon—especially if it's something sharp or mechanized like a vibrator, which will likely burn your inner tissues before the doctor can remove it and shut it off. Performers run risks every time they shove something like this up their asses, all covered in slippery lube and difficult to hang onto, though it's true that these professional performers have highly trained muscles from years of inserting and expelling objects. Also, starlets seem to be able to just take a toy, penis, or huge object in their asses without any warm-up. The directors never show you that the performers spend time relaxing their anuses with lubed fingers and toys, or that some even prepare the night before a shoot. To insert anything without preparation and lube will rip the dry, thin tissues of the anus, causing unbelievable pain and bleeding. Don't try it at home.

Another unsafe portrayal of sex in porn is the nonexistence of lube. As if by magic, the penis or sex toy slides right into the vagina or anus, or alternatively a little licking precedes a fast anal penetration. Lubrication is used, but is never shown to an audience that the filmmakers assume don't want to see lube. The skyrocketing sales of lube to a hungry, deliciously slippery populace shows that people who are having sex are finding lube necessary and sexy as hell (to apply and use), so it's puzzling that pornographers haven't clued into this obvious fact. Dry sex, especially anal sex, increases the chances of disease and virus transmission, plus it doesn't feel an eighth as good as sex with slick sex parts.

Nonlubricated sex portrayals (anal and vaginal) compound viewer ignorance about pleasure and safety, and also intensify feelings of blame and inadequacy surrounding natural vaginal lubrication, which is neither a reliable means to measure arousal nor a sure thing to expect. Natural vaginal lubrication is subject to medication, vitamins, emotional state, and any number of health factors. In porn you'll see performers using saliva as lube, which is in most cases a misrepresentation of the fact that they have already applied lube out of a bottle. Also, saliva is no a substitute for lube, for it dries out in seconds, doesn't provide the slip necessary for extended in-and-out thrusting, and is in every other way unsuitable for anal penetration. Plus, if you've ever tried it, you know what a poor lubricant saliva alone is. Don't believe the hype.

Read more about the testing precautions taken—or not taken—by performers for STDs and HIV/AIDS in Chapter 5, "Common Concerns About Content." Remember that a condom worn by the male partner significantly reduces chances of spreading STDs and HIV/AIDS for both anal/vaginal penetration and fellatio, while a dental dam (a thin sheet of latex) or plastic wrap barrier prevents fluid transmission during cunnilingus and rimming. The following charts show the diseases for which an individual is at risk when engaging in common porn sex acts without safer-sex barriers such as condoms or dental dams.

Porn Safer Sex Charts

Unprotected Fellatio (Giving)

HIGH RISK	MODERATE RISK	NO RISK	N/A
Gonorrhea	Chlamydia	Hepatitis A	Bacterial vaginosis
Hepatitis B	HIV	Hepatitis C	Vaginitis
Herpes	Lice/scabies		
Syphilis	HPV		

Unprotected Fellatio (Getting)

HIGH RISK	MODERATE RISK	NO RISK	N/A
Gonorrhea	Chlamydia	Hepatitis A	Bacterial vaginosis
Herpes	HPV	Hepatitis C	Vaginitis
Syphilis	HIV		
	Hepatitis B		
	Lice/scabies		

Unprotected Cunnilingus (Giving)

HIGH RISK	MODERATE RISK	NO RISK	N/A
Gonorrhea	HIV	Chlamydia	Bacterial vaginosis
Herpes	HPV	Hepatitis A	Vaginitis
Syphilis	Lice/scabies	Hepatitis B	
		Hepatitis C	

Unprotected Cunnilingus (Getting)

HIGH RISK	MODERATE RISK	NO RISK	N/A
Gonorrhea	Chlamydia	Hepatitis A	Bacterial vaginosis
Herpes	HPV	Hepatitis B	Vaginitis
Syphilis	Lice/scabies	Hepatitis C	
		HIV	

Porn Safer Sex Charts

Unprotected Rimming (Giving)

HIGH RISK	MODERATE RISK	NO RISK	N/A
Gonorrhea	Chlamydia	None	Bacterial vaginosis
Hepatitis A	Hepatitis C		Vaginitis
Hepatitis B	HIV		
Herpes	Lice/scabies		
HPV			
Syphilis			

Unprotected Rimming (Getting)

HIGH RISK	MODERATE RISK	NO RISK	N/A
Gonorrhea	Chlamydia	Hepatitis A	Bacterial vaginosis
Hepatitis B	Hepatitis C		Vaginitis
Herpes	HPV		
Syphilis	HIV		
	Lice/scabies		

Anal-to-Oral Contact (Penis or Sex Toy)

HIGH RISK	MODERATE RISK	NO RISK	N/A
Gonorrhea	HIV	Lice/scabies	Bacterial vaginosis
Hepatitis A	Chlamydia		Vaginitis
Hepatitis B	Hepatitis C		
Herpes			
HPV			
Syphilis			

Sharing Sex Toys

HIGH RISK	MODERATE RISK	NO RISK	N/A
Chlamydia	Bacterial vaginosis	None	None
Gonorrhea	Hepatitis A		
Hepatitis B	Hepatitis C		
HIV	Herpes		
Syphilis	HPV		
	Lice/scabies		
	Vaginitis		

Deep Kissing

HIGH RISK	MODERATE RISK	NO RISK	N/A
None	Gonorrhea	Chlamydia	Bacterial vaginosis
	Hepatitis B	Hepatitis A	Vaginitis
	Herpes	Hepatitis C	
	HPV	HIV	
	Syphilis	Lice/scabies	

Dry Kissing

HIGH RISK	MODERATE RISK	NO RISK	N/A
None	None	Bacterial vaginosis	None
		Chlamydia	
		Gonorrhea	
		Hepatitis A	
		Hepatitis B	
		Hepatitis C	
		Herpes	
		HIV	
		HPV	
		Lice/scabies	
		Syphilis	

Porn Safer Sex Charts

*Ejaculation in Eyes**

HIGH RISK	MODERATE RISK	NO RISK	N/A
Chlamydia	HIV	Hepatitis A	Bacterial vaginosis
Gonorrhea	HPV	Hepatitis C	Vaginitis
Hepatitis B			Lice/scabies
Herpes			
Syphilis			

* Chlamydia, gonorrhea, and syphilis will cause conjunctivitis.

Ejaculation on Exterior of Female Genitals

HIGH RISK	MODERATE RISK	NO RISK	N/A
Gonorrhea	Chlamydia	None	Bacterial vaginosis
Hepatitis A	Hepatitis C		Lice/scabies
Hepatitis B	HIV		Vaginitis
Herpes			
HPV			
Syphilis			

Ejaculation in Nose

HIGH RISK	MODERATE RISK	NO RISK	N/A
Chlamydia	HIV	None	Bacterial vaginosis
Gonorrhea	HPV		Hepatitis A
Hepatitis B			Hepatitis C
Herpes			Lice/scabies
Syphilis			Vaginitis

Unprotected Anal-to-Vaginal Contact

HIGH RISK	MODERATE RISK	NO RISK	N/A
Bacterial vaginosis	Hepatitis C	None	Lice/scabies
Chlamydia			
Gonorrhea			
Hepatitis A			
Hepatitis B			
Herpes			
HIV			
HPV			
Syphilis			

Unprotected Penis/Vagina Sex

HIGH RISK	MODERATE RISK	NO RISK	N/A
Bacterial vaginosis	Hepatitis A	None	None
Chlamydia	Hepatitis C		
Gonorrhea			
Hepatitis B			
Herpes			
HIV			
HPV			
Lice/scabies			
Syphilis			

Unprotected Anal Sex

HIGH RISK	MODERATE RISK	NO RISK	N/A
Gonorrhea	None	Bacterial vaginosis	None
Hepatitis B		Chlamydia	
Hepatitis C		Hepatitis A	
Herpes			
HIV			
HPV			
Lice/scabies			
Syphilis			

Porn Terminology and Sex Act Glossary

69 (sixty-nine) When two people give simultaneous oral sex to one another, creating a "69" shape.

AC/DC Bisexual male; also, Australian rock band.

All-Natural Indicates when starlets have natural, unenhanced breasts, that is, no plastic surgery or overstuffed boob jobs.

Analingus Licking around the anus or inserting the tongue into the anus. Also known as "rimming."

ATM Abbreviated term for "ass to mouth." When a finger, penis, or sex toy is inserted anally, then orally without stopping to clean it off. Common in porn but in real life will likely give you hepatitis A.

Autoerotic Asphyxiation Method of heightening arousal from lack of oxygen, by strangling. Also known as "choking."

Autoerotica Self-induced arousal from fantasies, pornographic materials, or other erotic aids.

Back Spackle In doggie-style position, pulling out and ejaculating onto the back or buttocks.

Ballstretching Wrapping the scrotum with some kind of leather strap tightly and pulling down with increasing pressure, the goal being the stretchee's pleasure. Read more about it in Hardy Haberman's *Family Jewels*.

B/D (*see* S/M)

Bear A large, hairy, gay man. Usually friendly.

Bisexual Individuals who are attracted to both men and women. In porn, it refers to titles that depict two men with one woman, and the men have sex with each other in addition to the female (unlike threesomes in straight porn where the men are homophobic). The men are usually gay porn actors.

Blood Sports Sexual activity involving the drawing of blood or piercing. This is rarely represented in porn.

Body Bag A fully enclosed, specially made rubber bag into which an S/M "bottom" is sealed. Used in restriction or "mummification" games, and sometimes for punishment. You'd better believe these bags are very expensive, and only available through specialty S/M boutiques.

Bondage Restricting a partner's movement with ropes, leather cuffs, handcuffs, or other devices. Usually in an S/M context, though seldom shown in porn along with sex.

Bottom A submissive in S/M.

Boy In role-playing, a "daddy's" submissive. Can be either male or female.

Brown Showers Sex play involving defecation.

Bukkake Supposedly an ancient custom hailing from parts of Japan where, as punishment or a form of humiliation for an adulterous woman, ten to a hundred men gather around and ejaculate onto her. Whether truly a tradition or not, or a figment of the adult industry, it's now a trendy staple on the fringes of American porn. Where the ejaculations end up depends on the filmmaker: face, whole body, mouth—in one case, the actress wears a dog cone. The actress never has intercourse with the men, and the come is dealt with in creative, if stomach-churning, ways.

Butch A lesbian who cultivates and identifies with her masculine traits.

CBT Short for "cock and ball torture." Refers to pleasurable—and painful—torment of a man's cock and balls, in the context of S/M.

Classics These are films made in the 1970s and 1980s, though the term usually refers to famous or notorious older films such as *Deep Throat, Devil in Miss Jones,* and *Behind the Green Door.*

Cock Ring A leather, neoprene, metal, or rubber ring placed around a man's balls and cock to apply a pleasurable restriction to the whole package. Many men enjoy the sensation of pressure, as the cock ring can aid in restricting blood flow to and from the penis and make a stiffer hard-on, sometimes also helping them maintain an erection for longer than usual. Not reliable for creating an erection, or for erectile dysfunction. Also enjoyed on nonerect members.

Contract Girl A female performer chosen for new or reigning superstardom by a big production company to go under contract for a term of time or number of movies. The production company then focuses new releases and marketing campaigns around the starlet. For more background, see Chapter 5.

Couples Porn, or The Couples Market Loose term for porn that pornographers think couples and women categorically want to watch. Assumes an interest in "softer" porn (that is, no rough stuff), but can indicate a high-budget, well-written, plot-driven film.

Cowgirl Woman sitting on man's lap while having sex, facing him. Also known as "woman on top."

Cream Pie An actress with come visibly dripping from her vagina or anus.

Cub A smaller, young submissive who likes bears.

Cum Spelling variation derivative of the adult industry; term for ejaculate.

DA (Double Anal) Two penises in one ass at the same time.

Discipline The "D" in BDSM. The act of punishing a submissive.

Docking Insertion of the penis into the foreskin of another man.

Doggie Style Also known as "doggie." One participant is on all fours, and penetrated from behind.

DP (Double Penetration) In porn, a "double penetration" refers to two men penetrating one woman simultaneously in the ass and vagina. In gay porn, the term refers to two men penetrating one man in the ass simultaneously.

D/S (see S/M)

DV (Double Vaginal) Two penises in the vagina at the same time.

DVDA The name of South Park creators Trey Parker and Matt Stone's band. Is it really possible? You tell me.

Edge Play S/M that involves a real risk of injury or death, such as electrical or breath play. Also refers to S/M that pushes the boundaries of psychological comfort, such as humiliation scenes.

Educational Videos that have an educational aspect but feature explicit demonstrations or hard-core sex, or both.

Enema, Enema Play An enema is an anal douche, or a means of filling the lower colon with water to flush and clean the lower colon and anal canal. Enema kits are sold in pharmacies. Porn stars use enemas regularly, especially before scenes involving anal sex. This is how porn stars mini- mize contracting hepatitis A when inserting penises and sex toys from anus to mouth, though it is not a surefire way of preventing the virus. (And because it is a virus, it never goes away.) Enema play is featured in extreme fetish videos, where participants, usually women, have enemas administered as punishment, or play with them sexually.

European Porn made in Europe, notable for the natural beauty or attractiveness of the performers and their mature, though deliciously uninhibited, approach to sex.

Feature Porn with a plot.

Femme A lesbian who cultivates and identifies with her femininity, often enjoying high heels, lipstick, and other stylistic accoutrements.

Fingercuffing When a woman or man is penetrated vaginally or anally while performing fellatio on another male.

FIP (Fake Internal Pop Shot) The cable version of an orgasmic climax in which both partners simply shudder violently, faking orgasm.

Fisting Insertion of all four fingers and the thumb into vagina or anus, which then curl into a small, loose fist. This is a sexual practice enjoyed by those who like the feeling of being "full" or stretched. While practiced by many regular folks, it may be considered obscene to depict.

Fluffer A woman or man used to stimulate male talent through oral sex before they go on camera. Reports on whether fluffers still exist in porn conflict greatly.

FTM A female-to-male transsexual.

Gang Bang When four or more guys have sex with one woman at the same time. The first marathon gang bang was the Annabel Chong 251, where she had sex with 251 men. To date the largest gang bang was the Houston 620. It was originally called the Houston 500, but the recipient was determined to make a record no one could break, so, what the hell, added another 120 guys.

Gape, Gapes, Gaping Term for when the pussy or ass is stretched or held open to create a hole you can see into. Currently a trendy fetish in the all-sex genre.

Glory Hole A hole in a partition or wall of an arcade booth that allows a person on the other side to engage in a sexual activity; a penis is inserted on one side, and you can figure out the rest. Sometimes a hole in a bathroom stall used for sex, oral and anal. There is a great glory hole scene in *Bad Wives*.

Golden Showers Also known as "pee play" or "pissing." Urinating onto another person for mutual sexual gratification.

Gonzo A porn genre where there is no plot and the person with the camera directs the action, occasionally getting involved and giving the viewer a first-person experience. Takes its name from Hunter S. Thompson's irreverent, improvised situational style of journalism.

Handkerchief Codes Gay leatherman and leatherdyke handkerchief color codes and methods of wearing them, used to identify sexual preferences.

Hard, Hard-core Refers to the explicit version of an adult film, with explicit penetration, genital close-ups, and ejaculation, as opposed to the "soft-core" version, edited for cable viewing.

Harness Body harnesses used in BDSM suspension, or a strap-on harness worn to wear a dildo used for penetrating a partner.

Hedgehog Ron Jeremy.

Hentai Explicit animated Japanese porn that typically includes use of taboo subjects such as sibling incest, transsexual sex, or sex with animals or with supernatural monsters, gods, and ghosts.

Huffing A blow job; for example, "huffing cock."

Independent Films that come from independent distribution sources and small production companies. Can include films from individuals, woman-owned sex toy companies, and so on.

Inflation A fetish for growth of particular body parts, such as breasts or labia. Outlets are found in big-bust films, or S/M films where breast inflation is temporarily induced with saline injections. Also in fetish porn where a rubber isolation suit (or body bag) is worn and inflated with air.

IP Internal "pop shot" or ejaculation.

Junk N Da Trunk A big butt.

Kegel Named after a male gynecologist, one Dr. Kegel, who publicized the self-named Kegel exercise. Involves the flexing of the pelvic muscles that control orgasm and inner vaginal muscles. Usually used for toning and for tightening.

Lesbian, Girl–Girl, or All-Girl In mainstream porn, a film that is all women, though the women performing are seldom lesbians.

Looner A balloon fetishist. Looners use large, sturdy balloons in sex play with partners, but more often prefer simply humping the balloons themselves. There are two groups of looners: poppers, who prefer that the balloons eventually pop, and nonpoppers, who do not.

Mish, or Missionary (Position) Sexual position supposedly touted by missionaries and clergy as the proper position for intercourse, male superior. Recipient is on their back with legs spread, penetrator is on top.

Money Shot Male ejaculation captured on film; volume and distance are highly prized.

MTF A male-to-female transsexual.

Mullet Haircut popularized by 1980s glam and metal bands in which the top and sides are short, while the back is grown long, creating a frightening waterfall effect. Worn by many lesbians (and professional wrestlers) well into the 1990s and even up to the present. See www.mulletsgalore.com.

Mummification In BDSM a person subjected to mummification is completely wrapped up, with breathing holes or tubes. This practice enhances sensations of constriction, or helplessness, depending on how the preplanned BDSM scene is constructed. Saran Wrap is a common mummification aid.

Nipple Clamps or Clips Metal, clothespin, or rubber clips or clamps that attach to the nipples and provide a constant pinching sensation, producing simultaneous pain and pleasure. Especially intense when removed.

Pearl Necklace Term referring to ejaculation onto a woman's neckline and breasts, thereby simulating a string of pearls.

Pocket Rocket A type of small vibrator with a single hard, bumpy end that is popular with porn stars and used frequently in porn.

Ponyboy/Ponygirl Intense and specialized role-play where the submissive assumes the role of horse or pony, and is trained or used by a trainer. Ponies can be male or female, and the costly gear can range from custom-made human saddles and bridles to horsehair butt plugs. Not for folks who only earn minimum wage.

Pop Shot When a man ejaculates, and it is caught on film.

Pro-Am Short for "professional/amateur," describing participants who are new to adult films having sex with professionals, but can also include women who are not really new to adult but are having a first-time experience on camera, or are experienced in adult but are new to a series. These films are all-sex, no plot, usually shot gonzo-style.

Raincoater Industry term for the person producers believe buys their hard-core pornography; term does not include women or couples. Slightly demeaning term, indicating desperate men wearing raincoats to hide their erections.

Reverse Cowgirl Woman on top, facing away from man while having sex, ideal for spread-wide hard-core shots because it provides the maximum view of penetration.

Reverse Cowgirl's Blog Witty Susannah Breslin's web log, "Wherein a writer attempts to justify the enormity of her porn collection." See "More Choice Clickables" in Chapter 14, "Resources."

Reverse Gang Bang When four or more women have sex with one man. I had hoped this would be a group of women pushing a guy around and demanding that he make them come until they were through with him, but I was sadly disappointed. The male is the active party, with all the females receptive to his busy, sweaty humping.

Rim Job, Rimming Licking around the anus; *see* Analingus.

Scene (1) A segment of sex in an adult film; (2) a negotiated and planned enactment of S/M activities.

S/M Includes B/D (bondage and discipline), S/M (sadomasochism), and D/S (dominance and submission). These practices cover spanking, whipping, caning, restraint with ropes and leather, erotic torture with everything from clothespins to mild electricity, and "forced" submission, or training. Some S/M activities take place in professional dungeons, and all occur between consenting adults who have negotiated the scene beforehand. S/M films seldom contain sex.

Snowballing The term for swapping ejaculate from one mouth to another, or kissing someone after they have received a mouthful of come.

Soft, Soft-core Term referring to the non-explicit version of a porn film (edited for cable viewing), or any film that implies but does not show penetration, genital close-ups, or ejaculation.

Specialty Porn When porn is labeled "specialty," it usually contains a sex act or falls into a category outside conventional heterosexual tastes—though that can cover ground that many find disturbing or even shocking. Sometimes S/M is lumped into this category. Specialty can include transsexuals, fat folks, the elderly, or midgets; fetishes such as foot, breast, panties, or lactation; pregnant women; hairy women; and more.

Speculum A duck-bill-shaped device that a gynecologist uses to spread open the walls of the vagina to see the cervix. Used in sex education films and S/M films.

Spooning Sexual position in which the penetrator cradles the recipient from behind.

St. Andrews Cross In S/M, a giant X-shaped cross on which submissives are strapped in place.

Strap-On A harness worn on the pelvis to hold a dildo erect from the pubic mound for penetration of a partner. Worn, received, and loved by all genders.

Suitcase Pimp A starlet's unemployed boyfriend or husband, generally abusive and annoying, who carries her suitcase onto a film set. Usually seen talking into a cell phone trying to look important, and acting as her "agent."

Teabagging Usually performed by dipping the testicles onto a participant's face, or specifically the mouth. Also sucking on a man's balls. Watch John Waters's *Pecker* for a hilarious demonstration—or three.

Transsexual, Tranny A person who identifies with and lives as a gender other than that assigned at birth. In porn, usually refers to someone in process of physically changing sexes, and generally refers to women transitioning from male bodies into female ones. "Tranny porn" features women with penises, usually fully functional, meaning they can achieve erections and ejaculate.

Twinkie, Twink A submissive, boyish gay male who receives penetration, hence the cream filling.

Voyeurism Arousal by watching others engaged in sexual activities.

Viagra A pharmaceutical aid created to treat male impotence. Viagra constricts the flow of blood in the penis, sustaining arousal and delaying ejaculation. Now the backbone, so to speak, of the porno biz.

Wall-to-Wall These videos are all-sex, no-plot. Usually a tape of sex scenes strung together loosely by a theme, such as amateurs, or focusing on a sex act, such as fellatio, or both, as in first-time anal sex.

Water Sports Urine fetishes, or arousal from sex play with urine. See Golden Showers.

Woman-Directed Films directed, and often written, by women (usually former performers). They tend to focus on female pleasure and enjoyment, have plenty of chemistry and higher production values.

Resources: Where to Buy and Rent Your Porn

Women-Friendly Adult Retail Stores, U.S.

Come Again Erotic Emporium

Woman-owned store with toys, books, videos and lingerie; it also has a book and fetish catalog. Opened by Helen Wolf in 1981.

353 E. 53rd St., New York, NY 10022

(212) 308-9394

www.comeagainnyc.com

Eve's Garden

Woman-focused store and catalog of toys, books, and videos. Nice, small handpicked selection of videos with women's pleasure in mind.
119 W. 57th St., Ste. #1201, New York, NY 10019
(212) 757-8651; (800) 848-3837
www.evesgarden.com

Good Vibrations

Pioneering the woman-owned, woman-focused sex shop since 1977, this store has grown to employ and serve all communities and orientations with the mission of promoting pleasure and accurate sex information. Staff is meticulously trained, and its Education department serves staff and customers and does outreach to health organizations. Mail-order catalog, website, and retail stores carry toys, books, videos, DVDs, safer-sex supplies, magazines, and comics. All products are individually selected and reviewed, and the stores offer ongoing after-hours classes. Dr. Carol Queen is the staff sexologist.
1210 Valencia St., San Francisco, CA 94110; (415) 974-8980
2504 San Pablo Ave., Berkeley, CA 94702; (510) 841-8987
1620 Polk St., San Francisco, CA 94109; (415) 345-0400
Mail order (800) 289-8423
www.goodvibes.com
(See "Online and Mail Order" and "Online Rentals" sections for more information.)

Grand Opening!

Retail store, website, and mail-order catalog of toys, books, safer-sex supplies, and carefully selected videos; store has classes and events, some taught and hosted by owner Kim Airs.
318 Harvard St., Ste. 32, Arcade Bldg., Coolidge Corner, Brookline, MA 02446
(617) 731-2626
8442 Santa Monica Blvd., Los Angeles (West Hollywood), CA 90069
(323) 848-6970
Mail order (877) 731-2626
www.grandopening.com

Pleasure Chest

Retail store, website (address and hours only, no online store—yet), and catalog of novelties, toys, videos, and clothing. They have a very friendly staff and a great selection of gay and straight videos.
7733 Santa Monica Blvd., West Hollywood, CA 90046
(323) 650-1022; (800) 75-DILDO
www.thepleasurechest.com

Purple Passion

Retail store and website of toys, books, videos, magazines, and fetish clothing and shoes, plus a full selection of S/M and bondage toys and accoutrements. Mainly geared toward BDSM shoppers. Their fine-tuned video selection specializes in S/M and fetishes such as rubber, corsets, and more.
211 West 20th St., New York, NY 10011; (212) 807-0486
www.purplepassion.com

Toys in Babeland

Retail store, website, and catalog of toys, books, videos, and safer-sex supplies. Women-owned and -operated, and open to all orientations. Their videos are handpicked and individually reviewed, and they boast a friendly, knowledgeable staff. Also offers in-store educational workshops.
707 E. Pike St., Seattle, WA 98122; (206) 328-2914
94 Rivington St., New York, NY 10002; (212) 375-1701
Mail order (800) 658-9119
www.babeland.com

A Woman's Touch

Feminist sex store offering toys, books, videos and safer-sex supplies. Its website has great advice columns, and the video selection is carefully categorized for easy decision-making. Especially notable is the separate sections for sexually explicit instructional videos (vs. non-explicit), and videos with real couples in them (vs. performers).
600 Williamson St., Madison, WI 53703
(608) 250-1928; (888) 6218880
www.a-womans-touch.com

Women-Friendly Adult Retail Stores, Canada

Come As You Are

No trip to Toronto is complete without visiting this community-oriented worker-owned co-op retail store, which also has a mail-order catalog and website. It sells toys, books, videos, safer-sex supplies, and educational resources, especially resources for the disabled. Products are handpicked and individually reviewed, and their video selection is excellent. Store offers educational workshops. *Nous offrons des services limités en français.*
701 Queen St. W., Toronto, ON, M6J 1E6, Canada
(877) 858-3160; (416) 504-7934
www.comeasyouare.com

Good For Her

Woman-focused retail store carries toys, books, videos, and erotic art; hosts sex workshops, all geared toward female pleasure. In addition to regular hours, store has women-only hours.
171 Harbord St., Toronto, ON, M5S 1H5, Canada
(877) 588-0900; (416) 588-0900
www.goodforher.com

Lovecraft

Retail stores and website offer toys, books, videos, and lingerie. Possibly the oldest women-owned sex shop in North America—open since 1972.
27 Yorkville Ave., Toronto, ON, M4W 1L1, Canada
416 923 7331
2200 Dundas St. East, Mississauga, ON, L4X 2V3, Canada
905 276 5772; (877) 923-7331
www.lovecraftsexshop.com

Women-Friendly Adult Retail Stores, Europe

Coco de Mer

23 Monmouth St., Covent Garden, London WC2, U.K.; 020 7836 8882
www.coco-de-mer.co.uk

SH!

A women's sex shop.
22 Coronet St., London N1 6HD, U.K.; 020 7613 0020
www.sh-womenstore.com

Online and Mail Order, General

Adam and Eve

Mail-order catalog and website of toys, books, videos, DVDs, safer-sex supplies, and lingerie, with a heterosexual focus—they have online personal ads for customers, the website has a Spanish option. They are the oldest mail order face of the mainstream adult industry and have consistently fought to uphold the rights for retailers to sell adult products. Their video selection is large, and their Nina Hartley collection is impressive. Be sure to "opt out" on allowing them to share your information.
P.O. Box 200, Carrboro, NC 27510
(800) 274-0333; (919) 644-1212
www.adameve.com

Adult DVD Empire

Gigantic selection of mainstream videos and DVDs, with a sister site specializing in gay titles. They have a strict privacy policy, and offer inexpensive bundled titles and free shipping specials. Most notable are the comprehensive customer reviews on all the titles they carry.
www.adultdvdempire.com
www.gaydvdempire.com

Adult Video Universe

Discount new adult DVDs for sale, and a pretty big selection at that. Also carries video games, music, and nonerotic movies. It does not sell your information to third parties, but be sure to opt out of promotions with third parties that they might send via email (unless you want them). Their customer reviews are very helpful, and often get right to the point. Customer service is available 9 A.M. to 5 P.M. ET, Mon.–Fri. (except holidays). 101 N. Plains Industrial Road, Wallingford CT 06492-2360
(800) 231-7937; (203) 294 1648
www.cduniverse.com

Astral Ocean Cinema/Asia Blue/Mind Candy Emporium

This fluid site is a virtual clearinghouse for videos that cater to specific fetishes and aim for a clientele with exclusive tastes. They specialize in titles you'd be hard-pressed to find at your local video store. They also carry more Asian titles than most retailers and feature online pay-per-view porn. www.astralocean.com

Blissbox

A London-based website and mail-order company that offers videos and DVDs, sex toys and accoutrements, and possibly one of the best adult video review databases around. The site is smooth, incredibly well designed, and easy on the eyes; provides fan information on porn stars and offers sex tips that are accurate and to the point. Videos and toys paired together are a perfect combination, and Blissbox knows it. The tone of the site is healthy, nonjudgmental, supportive, and encouraging. It has a strict and simple privacy policy. Customer service 10 A.M. to 7 P.M. Mon.–Fri., U.K. time zone. Phone line is for orders only, with a £2 surcharge. Mail order: The website has a printable order form, though please check currency conversion rates if ordering outside the U.K.
Blackdog (their mail order company name)
P.O. Box 34984, London SW6 4XT, U.K.
0845 450 6655
www.blissbox.com

Blowfish

Mail-order catalog and website of toys, books, videos, DVDs, safer-sex supplies, S/M gear, comics, and magazines. Features individual (and often hilarious) reviews of its products—most notably their terrific video collection—and a strict privacy policy.
P.O. Box 411290, San Francisco, CA 94141
(800) 325-2569; (415) 252-4340
www.blowfish.com

Cult Epics

This site is a find for people seeking to purchase sophisticated porn. Cult Epics offers vintage porn from the 1930s and 1940s restored on DVD—right along with Maria Beatty's black-and-white modern classics and many uncut (explicit) films by *Caligula* director Tinto Brass. They're also building their cult/horror sections. They often have shipping specials.
www.cultepics.com

Gamelink

Purchase or view adult videos online from Gamelink's exhaustive selection—though no rentals yet. Not only is its selection extensive in both videos and DVDs, but it also carries sex toys, leather goods, and more. Free shipping over set purchase amounts, discount clubs, and a strict privacy policy.
Gamelink, Inc.
537 Stevenson Street, Suite 100, San Francisco, CA 94103
(415) 575-9700
Mail order (800) 944-3933
www.gamelink.com

Good Vibrations

Promoting pleasure since 1977, Good Vibrations has a staff who are extensively trained and up-to-date on all things sex-related and are committed to dispensing accurate sex information about the products they sell. See "Retail Stores" for more information. Mail order is open 7 A.M. to 7 P.M., PT. Carol Queen is the staff sexologist. Strict privacy policy. (For retail information, see "Retail Stores" and "Online Rentals.")
938 Howard St., Ste. 101, San Francisco, CA 94103
(800) 289-8423; (415) 974-8980
www.goodvibes.com

Jaded Video

A homegrown-looking website belies the fact that this site has more than 42,000 adult videos and DVDs. They have extensive in-house reviews on select titles, and they carry videos that range from the standard adult title to the edgier and more extreme. Strict privacy policy, with good prices. Online purchase only.
www.jadedvideo.com

Lezlove Video

These guys aren't lesbians. But they have a huge—gigantic—catalog of all-girl and real lesbian videos and DVDs, all reviewed by in-house reviewers and customers. It looks like a cheesy guys-version-of-lesbians site, and it is, but scratch the surface and you'll find all kinds of amateur, vintage, independent, Japanese, and mainstream explicit lesbian-themed titles. Many of the male reviewers don't like to see the women play with dildos (!?), but a surprising number of real lesbians and dykes write reviews, too.
www.lezlovevideo.com

Toys in Babeland

Website, retail stores, and catalog of toys, books, videos, and safer-sex supplies. Women-owned and -operated, but open to all orientations. Strict privacy policy. (For retail information, see "Retail Stores.")
(800) 658-9119
www.babeland.com

Xandria Collection

Mail-order catalog and website of toys, books, videos, DVDs, leather, and lingerie. They have a nice mixture of women-focused, fetish, and gay male titles. Betty Dodson is on its advisory board. Xandria has a stringent privacy policy.
165 Valley Dr., Brisbane, CA 94005
(415) 468-3812; (800) 242-2823
www.xandria.com

Online Adult Video and DVD Rentals

Blue Door

Buy or rent adult videos, with a huge selection helpfully divided into understandable sections. Videos are rated for excitement and entertainment, and are individually reviewed by both staff and customers, making this site an excellent resource. Strict privacy policy.
ETP Inc.
P.O. Box 64378, Sunnyvale, CA 94089
(888) 922-4387
www.bluedoor.com

Adult DVD Overnight

A decent, though not exhaustive, selection of adult videos, this reputable site is affiliated with a nonerotic DVD rental site, but it has a great overview of titles. Free shipping, inexpensive per-rental charges rather than month-by-month plans, an easy-to-use website; also sells adult novelties. Has a strict privacy policy, so no film titles appear on your billing record, but does not ship outside the mainland U.S., and its search engine is very basic.
DVDOvernight, Inc.
P.O. Box 2716, Ventnor, NJ 08406
(877) DVD-1099
www.adultdvdovernight.com

Flicksmart

With a gigantic selection (more than 6,000 titles), no late fees, and several monthly plans—it's a pretty straightforward arrangement. It offers many genres and a mind-boggling list of production companies to search through. Doesn't sell your information, but be sure that you opt out of any promotional mailings when you set up your account (if you want).
FSO, LLC
3884 Schiff Dr., Las Vegas, NV 89103
(702) 365-0800
www.flicksmart.com

Good Vibrations

You can rent its entire video selection online or over the phone. See "Retail Stores" for more information.
938 Howard St., Ste. 101, San Francisco, CA 94103
(800) 289-8423; (415) 974-8980
www.goodvibes.com; http://rentals.goodvibes.com

Green Cine

A small DVD rental biz run out of good old San Francisco by totally nerdy film geeks, this site doesn't carry hard-core per se, but does carry every wacko retro sexploitation film you've never heard of. If you love cheesy sleazy titles that sound like *Revenge of the Cannibal Cheerleaders* or *Zombie Apocalypse of the Lesbian Vampires,* or any Roger Corman films, this is ground zero for cult nudie horror flicks that most mainstream rental places wouldn't touch. But that's not all. It also carries all kinds of foreign, independent, soft-core (some Radley Metzger), and offbeat theater releases. And all the profits go to various film foundations. Will send you promotional coupons, but won't do anything with your information without your permission. Offers five monthly membership plans that vary in price according to how many titles you want to rent at a time.
www.greencine.com

Sugar DVD

An enormous selection, lively customer reviews, no due dates or late fees, and five different rental plans to choose from. Has a privacy policy and won't sell, rent, or trade your customer information with anyone, yet will send you its offers and promotions via email and regular mail, as well as promotions with partnered businesses (unless you request otherwise).
Sugar DVD/Oddesse
P.O. Box 55878, Sherman Oaks, CA 91413
(323) 876-1681
www.sugarDVD.com

Video Takeout

A medium-sized selection of titles for rent, with zero late fees, but an odd rental plan where the price increases with the number of postage-paid mailers you want. Features a nice director search function, though no date of release or running time for the films, and their site is tricky to navigate. Good privacy policy.
www.videotakeout.com

WantedList.com

Wanted List has more than 6,000 videos and DVDs to choose from, and pricing plans that suit individual rental styles. Flat rates, no late fees, and free shipping. Has a strict privacy policy.
Customer Service
P.O. Box 8469, Van Nuys, CA 91409
www.wantedlist.com

Adult Video Resources and Reviews

Adult DVD Empire

Comprehensive customer reviews on all the titles they carry—which is a lot! An incredible resource if you want really detailed descriptions before you buy, and plenty of gay reviews on their gay site.
www.adultdvdempire.com
www.gaydvdempire.com

Adult DVD Talk

Lots of ratings and extensive reviews of adult DVD titles, with advanced searches and purchase price comparisons.
www.adultdvdtalk.com

DVD Talk

"The Blue Room: Intelligent Talk About Adult...." An excellent source for reviews on adult DVDs, and a division of Adult DVD Empire.
www.dvdtalk.com/adult/index.html

Internet Adult Film Database

No pictures, just accurate data on more than 40,000 titles and some 32,000 performers and directors, plus search matches that get as specific as performer-pairings in scenes.
www.iafd.com

PornoPopDVD

Reviews, news interviews, and on-the-set features, all about today's porn.
www.pornopopdvd.com

Search Extreme

What's not to love about an adult site where you can search for literally anything? Search by performer, title, even obscure fetishes—and learn a thing or two about these fetishes at the same time. Great site with in-house reviews, though the reviewers can be pretty crass.
www.searchextreme.com

Talking Blue

Although a little dated, this site has extensive bios on hundreds of male and female performers, with their full title lists.
www.talkingblue.com

• •

A Good Cause: AIM Healthcare

A NONPROFIT corporation created to care for the physical and emotional needs of sex workers and the people who work in the adult entertainment industry. Through HIV and STD testing and treatment, counseling, and support-group programs, the staff serves and cares for the sex worker community. Their goal is to provide health care for body, mind, emotion, and spirit. Its website has an invaluable wealth of information for performers, including the sexual health responsibilities of porn performers. It needs donations! Clinic hours 10 a.m. to 5:30 p.m., Mon.–Fri.; 1 to 5 p.m., Sat.; closed Sun.

AIM Health Care Foundation
14241 Ventura Blvd., Ste. 105
Sherman Oaks, CA 91423
(818) 981 5681 voice
(818) 981 3851 fax
www.aim-med.org

• •

Safer Sex Resources

American Social Health Association

P.O. Box 13827, Research Triangle Park, Durham, NC 27709
(919) 361-8400

Centers for Disease Control National AIDS Clearinghouse

P.O. Box 6003, Rockville, MD 20849
(800) 342-AIDS
www.cdcnac.com

Cetra Latex-Free Supplies

A product site for latex-free gear, catering mainly to the medical community (because so many medical professionals end up with latex allergies). Sells to individuals. Nice sitewide search.
(888) LATEX-NO; (510) 848-3345
www.latexfree.com

Condomania

Exhaustive site that sells virtually every condom under the sun, with fun facts, lots of condom information, and a helpful condom shopping guide.
(800) 9CONDOM; (800) 926-6366
www.condomania.com

Glyde Dams

Buy 'em here, by the dozen or in a party pack!
www.sheerglydedams.com

National AIDS Hotline

(800) 342-2437

National STD Hotline

(800) 227-8922

Planned Parenthood

(800) 230-PLAN

www.ppfa.org

Safer Sex Page

www.safersex.org

San Francisco Sex Information

Sex information and referral switchboard that provides free, nonjudgmental, anonymous, accurate information about anything sex related. Hours 3 P.M. to 9 P.M. PT, Mon.–Fri.. They also answer email questions.

(877) 472-7374; (415) 989-SFSI

www.sfsi.org

More Choice Clickables

Although many performers and adult resources have websites, I only list here my favorite, free websites—in addition to sites that do not have annoying pop-ups.

Adult Video News

Look out for one pop-up, but enjoy all the online content from the adult industry's slick, glossy trade magazine.

www.avn.com

Alison Tyler

Tyler's erotica is pretty much the hottest thing going on in the world of dirty, explicit fiction. I'm a big fan—her stories never fail to arouse and engage both my brain and my many other erogenous zones.

www.prettythingspress.com

AltSex

Information about all aspects of BDSM.
www.altsex.org

Andrew Blake

Fans of Blake will enjoy his tasteful website, and fans of his starlets will like the merchandise.
www.andrewblake.com

Anna Span

This sexy British woman started shooting porn films after graduating from Central St. Martin School of Art and Design with a Fine Arts degree in Film and Video. In her dissertation, "Towards A New Pornography," she explores the female perspective on porn. Span believes porn is an excellent genre, considering it one of the last underdeveloped and underexplored areas of film. She is the author of *Erotic Home Videos: Create Your Own Adult Films*.
www.easyote.co.uk

Annie Sprinkle

Annie is awesome! This woman went from naïve starlet to sex-positive porn goddess and beyond to the realm of spiritual sex coach and internationally acclaimed performance artist. Watch her great video, *Annie Sprinkle's Herstory of Porn,* and visit this gorgeous site belonging to a woman who has changed the way we look at women in porn.
www.anniesprinkle.org

Asia Carrera's XXX Buttkicking Homepage

Carrera's homepage is all that. This adult star has the brains to back it all up, and you can tell it on the site she built. Lots of good free stuff.
www.asiacarrera.com

Betty Dodson

The inimitable Dodson's site—full of information.
www.bettydodson.com

Black Mirror Productions

Joe Gallant's website, featuring all his extremely edgy, kinky, anything-goes art-fueled porn adventures.
www.blackmirror.com

Buttman

With porn director John "Buttman" Stagliano, it's all about the booty. If you like backsides, anal sex in all its permutations, and women who like it too, any film by Buttman is a gold mine. Stagliano has done for women's asses what Russ Meyer did for women's breasts—elevated them to objects of worship. This is his site, a shrine to ass and info HQ on his videos.
www.buttman.com

Carol Queen

The Queen of Hearts herself: pioneer, sex educator, sexual revolutionary, advice columnist, and pleasure activist. Absolutely beautiful site.
www.carolqueen.com

Chloe XXX

Very slick and in-depth site for one of the most beautiful and intelligent women in porn, Chloe. Beware of pop-ups, though.
www.chloexxx.com

Cleis Press

Cleis has published groundbreaking, informative, and controversial books about sex and politics since 1980. The publisher of this book, Cleis also has a great website showcasing its latest award-winning erotica, all its sex guidebooks, and Midnight Editions, its incredible consciousness-raising human rights books.
www.cleispress.com

Cleo Dubois

The online home of Cleo and Sybil Holiday, BDSM educators and professional dominants. Info on Cleo's videos, workshops and classes, and empowering words for those interested in BDSM.
www.sm-arts.com

Cupcake

She's so cute, she's so—naughty! I can't get enough of this softcore site that features schoolgirl Cupcake in adventures with pastries, "furries," balloons, spankings, messy food, and more.
www.sugarandspice.org

Daze Reader

A terrific site for keeping up with sex in the news—I visit daily.
www.dazereader.com

Dr. Ducky Doolittle: The Site of Sexual Curiosities

Sexy, brainy, and a fetish model? Wow, what a combo! Ducky teaches sex ed classes, dresses like a naughty clown, and sits in cakes—all with a provocative take on art and culture. Her site is full of fun, titillation (mmm, Duckycam) and sex ed resources.
www.drducky. com

The Extra Action Marching Band

Over thirty members in various states of undress, cross-dress and egress comprise this renegade marching band, complete with a full horn section, drum corps, pep squad dressed as kinky cheerleaders and a flag team of men and women who perform overtly sexual, explicit choreographed routines. What they do to music is simply pornographic.
www.extra-action.com

Fatale Media

The makers of some of the finest independent lesbian porn available, they carry many lesbian classics. Nan Kinney, one of the founding publishers of *On Our Backs* magazine, is the president of Fatale Media and producer of Fatale videos. They are primarily geared toward lesbians, yet count among their viewers "other adventurous souls." One of their bestselling releases is *Bend Over Boyfriend*.
www.fatalemedia. com

Furniture Porn

Hot chair-on-chair action, kinky recliners, all-amateur seating, and virile overstuffed armchairs await. Your living room will never look the same—it'll look sexier.
www.furnitureporn.com

Jane's Net

Reviewers cull oodles of sex-related and alternative lifestyle sites and list them with aplomb.
www.janesguide.com

Joseph Kramer's New School of Erotic Touch

A resource guide to the best videos on erotic touch. The creators of this site have screened over 400 videos in the development of their curriculum. The New School of Erotic Touch offers holistic classes with a spiritual approach.
www.eroticmassage.com

Libido Magazine

Once a tastefully compiled print magazine dedicated to erotica, articles and erotic art, *Libido* now lives online. They have a fabulous art gallery, and the site has in-depth information on their videos.
www.libidomag.com

Lou Paget

Sex educator and best-selling author Lou Paget's web site offers her own books, a selection of handpicked sex toys, and more. Hardworking Paget is dedicated to finding quality sex gear for couples and providing accurate sex information, and her sex seminars are highly rated. Heterosexual focus.
www.loupaget.com

Maria Beatty

Her independent S/M films are breathtaking, winning awards at film festivals, and her site is a feast for the eyes. See what's new, view stills, and more.
www.bleuproductions.com

Nina Hartley

Possibly the most beloved adult star of all time, Hartley is an advocate of sex education and free speech, and she has a beautiful site. Unfortunately most of it is for paying customers, but you can read her online journal and enjoy other neat stuff for free.
www.nina.com

Pervgrrl

Part of the Cyberdyke network, this site, which is dedicated to queer grrrl pervs, is beautifully designed; full of articles, erotica, links, and resources; and as hot as your daddy's engineer boots. For it, "Anything bordering on vanilla and 'normal' is terrifying and dirty and will be hidden from sight immediately."
www.pervgrrrl.org

Pornblography

A female publicist for the adult industry has a web log that's smart, funny, scathing, and always offering interesting perspectives on the adult industry from the inside.
www.pornblography.com

PornOrchestra

This somewhat spontaneously assembled twenty-five-plus member orchestra, complete with an authentic conductor, performs live (and lively) reinterpreted porn scores in movie theaters and art galleries while selected scenes from porn movies play. They perhaps sum up the conundrum of porn auteurs vs. viewers with their statement claiming that porn music is a "complicated genre that has taken its share of scorn, from adult film producers who refuse to pay it any mind to legions of consumers who instinctively snap the sound off after pressing "play."
www.thewrongelement.com/pornorchestra

Queer Net

Discussion lists galore for the lesbian, gay, bisexual, transgender, and S/M communities—you can even start your own!
www.queernet.org

The Reverse Cowgirl's Blog

Smarty-pants and professional porn pundit Susannah Breslin's web log, "Wherein a writer attempts to justify the enormity of her porn collection." Breslin is a journalist who has covered porn for many years, and her web log is updated frequently and with flair.
blogs.salon.com/0001437/

Scarlet Letters

Webzine of articles, erotica, and more.
www.scarletletters.com

Scarleteen

Cute, smart and hip webzine of sex information geared toward teen women.
www.scarleteen.com

SIECUS
(Sexuality Information and Education Council of the United States)

A national nonprofit organization that develops, collects, and disseminates information on sex, promotes sex education, and advocates individual choice.
130 W. 42nd St., Ste. 350, New York, NY 10036
(212) 819-9770
www.siecus.org

Sinclair Intimacy Institute

Dedicated to sex education, this company is dedicated to helping hetero-sexual couples better their relationships, and they do so by making oodles of sex ed videos.
www.bettersex.com

SIR Video

Two amazing women run this porn production company—the stunning Shar Rednour and the hot-to-trot Jackie Strano. This butch–femme team makes educational how-to videos for all orientations, plus all-dyke, all-sex porn that tops the charts and wins awards.
www.sirvideo.com

Thomas Roche

One of my favorite erotica authors, Roche can actually make a crime-noir erotica short story sexually graphic and laugh-out-loud funny. He's a very bad man who needs to be punished by a gang of cranky women in Catholic schoolgirl uniforms.
www.thomasroche.org

Tiny Nibbles

My very own site, which is spanked into shape every chance I can get my hands on its quivering little pages. Articles, porn reviews, toy reviews, orally fixated erotica, recommended reading, latest news, and more!
www.tinynibbles.com

Tristan Taormino

The creator of *The Ultimate Guide to Anal Sex for Women* book and video(s) has a site with personals, commerce, links to her *Village Voice* columns, and details about her new products.
www.puckerup.com

Venus or Vixen?

Read some smut! Cara Bruce's fun-filled webzine with articles, erotica, reviews, and more.
www.venusorvixen.com

References

Black, Andy. *Necronomicon 1: The Journal of Horror and Erotic Cinema*. London: Creation Books, 1996.

Brame, Gloria. *Come Hither: A Common Sense Guide*. New York: A Fireside Book, Simon & Schuster, 2000.

Brent, Steve, and Elizabeth Brent (contributor). *The Couple's Guide to the Best Erotic Videos*. New York: St. Martin's Griffen Press, 1997.

Bruce, Cara, and Lisa Motanarelli, Ph.D. *The First Year: Hepatitis C*. New York: Marlowe, 2002.

Burana, Lily. *Strip City: A Stripper's Farewell Journey Across America*. New York: Talk/Mirimax, 2001.

Califia, Patrick. *Public Sex: The Culture of Radical Sex*, 2d ed. San Francisco: Cleis Press, 2000.

———. *Sensuous Magic: A Guide for Adventurous Couples*. San Francisco: Cleis Press, 2001.

————. *Speaking Sex to Power*. San Francisco: Cleis Press, 2003.

Cohen, Angela, and Sarah Fox Gardner. *The Wise Woman's Guide to Erotic Videos: 300 Sexy Videos for Every Woman and Her Lover*. New York: Broadway Books, 1997.

Delacoste, Frédérique, and Priscilla Alexander. *Sex Work: Writings by Women in the Sex Industry*. San Francisco: Cleis Press, 1997.

Dodson, Betty. *Sex for One: The Joy of Selfloving*. New York: Crown Publications, 1997.

Gach, Michael Reed, Ph.D. *Acupressure for Lovers*. New York: Bantam Books, Bantam Doubleday Dell Publishing Group, 1997.

Gittler, Ian. *Pornstar*. New York: Simon & Schuster, 1999.

Goldstone, Stephen E., M.D. *The Ins and Outs of Gay Sex: A Medical Handbook for Men*. New York: Dell Publishing, Random House, 1999.

Haines, Staci. *The Survivor's Guide to Sex*. San Francisco: Cleis Press, 1999.

Heiman, Julia, Ph.D., and Joseph LoPiccolo, Ph.D. *Becoming Orgasmic*. New York: Simon & Schuster, 1988.

Holliday, Jim. *Only the Best*. Van Nuys, CA: Cal Vista Direct Publishing, 1986.

Janus, S. S., and C. L. Janus. *The Janus Report on Sexual Behavior*. New York: Wiley, 1993.

Joannides, Paul. *The Guide to Getting It On!* Waldport, OR: Goofy Foot Press, 2000.

Johnson, Merri Lisa (ed.). *Jane Sexes It Up*. New York: Four Walls Eight Windows, 2002.

Lerman, Evelyn. *Safer Sex: The New Morality*. Buena Park, CA: Morning Glory Press, 2000.

Levine, Judith. *Harmful to Minors*. Minneapolis, MN: University of Minnesota Press (Trd.), 2002.

Loftus, David. *Watching Sex: How Men Really Respond to Pornography*. New York: Thunder's Mouth Press, 2002.

Lotney, Karlyn. *The Ultimate Guide to Strap-On Sex*. San Francisco: Cleis Press, 2000.

Masters, W. H., V. E. Johnson, and R. C. Kolodny. *Human Sexuality*. Boston: Little, Brown, 1995.

————. *Masters and Johnson on Sex and Human Loving*. Boston: Little, Brown, 1985.

Matrix, Cherie (ed.). *Tales from the Clit: A Female Experience on Pornography*. San Francisco: AK Press, 1996.

McCarty, John. *The Sleaze Merchants: Adventures in Exploitation Filmmaking*. New York: St. Martin's Griffin Press, 2000.

McIlvenna, Ted, Clark Taylor, and the Institute for the Advanced Study of Human Sexuality. *The Complete Guide to Safer Sex*. New York: Barricade Books, 1999.

Men's Fitness Magazine, with John and Beth Tomkiw. *Total Sex: Men's Fitness Magazine's Complete Guide to Everything Men Need to Know and Want to Know About Sex*. New York: Harper Perennial, Harper Collins Publishers, 1999.

Milsten, Richard, M.D., and Julian Slowinski, Psy.D. *The Sexual Male: Problems and Solutions*. New York: W. W. Norton, 1999.

Morin, Jack, Ph.D. *The Erotic Mind*. New York: Harper Perennial, Harper Collins Publishers, 1995.

Petersen, James R., and Hugh M. Hefner. *The Century of Sex: Playboy's History of the Sexual Revolution, 1900–1999*. New York: Grove Press, 1999.

Poitras, Gilles. *Anime Essentials: Every Thing a Fan Needs to Know*. Berkeley, CA: Stone Bridge Press, 2001.

Queen, Carol. *Exhibitionism for the Shy*. San Francisco: Down There Press, 1995.

————. *Real Live Nude Girl: Chronicles of Sex-Positive Culture*. San Francisco: Cleis Press, 2002.

Rimmer, Robert H. The *X-Rated Videotape Guide*. New York: Harmony Books, Crown Publishers, 1984, 1986.

Rodgers, Joann Ellison. *Sex: The Natural History of a Behavior*. New York: W. H. Freeman, 2001.

Schlosser, Eric. *Reefer Madness: Sex, Drugs and Cheap Labor in the American Black Market*. New York: Houghton Mifflin, 2003.

Shakespeare, Tom, Kath Gillespie-Sells, Dominic Davies. *The Sexual Politics of Disability*. New York: Continuum, 1996.

Sheiner, Marcy. *Sex for the Clueless*. New York: Citadel Press, 2001.

Skee, Mickey. *The Best of Gay Adult Videos 1998: Mickey Skee's Dirty Dozens*. Laguna Hills, CA: Companion Press, 1998.

Span, Anna. *Erotic Home Videos: Create Your Own Adult Films*. London: Carlton, 2002.

Sprinkle, Annie. *Annie Sprinkle: Post Porn Modernist*. San Francisco: Cleis Press, 1998.

Stoller, Robert J., M.D. *Porn: Myths for the Twentieth Century*. New Haven and London: Yale University Press, 1991.

Stoller, Robert J., and I. S. Levine. *Coming Attractions: The Making of an X-Rated Video*. New Haven and London: Yale University Press, 1996.

Taormino, Tristan. *The Ultimate Guide to Anal Sex for Women*. San Francisco: Cleis Press, 1998.

Turner, Grady T., Martin Duberman, and Joan Nestle. *NYC Sex: How New York Transformed Sex in America*. New York: Scala Books, 2002.

Tyler, Parker. *Sex in Films*. New York: Carol Publishing Group, 1993.

Walker, Mitch. *Men Loving Men: A Gay Sex Guide and Consciousness Book*. San Francisco: Gay Sunshine Press, 1997.

Williams, Linda. *Hard Core: Power, Pleasure and the "Frenzy of the Visible."* Berkeley: University of California Press, 1999.

Winks, Cathy. *The Good Vibrations Guide: Adult Videos*. San Francisco: Down There Press, 1998.

Winks, Cathy, and Anne Semans. *The Good Vibrations Guide to Sex*, 3rd ed. San Francisco: Cleis Press, 1997, 2002.

Wolfe, Daniel. *Men Like Us: The GMHC Complete Guide to Gay Men's Sexual, Physical, and Emotional Well-Being*. New York: Ballantine Books, 2000.

Zilbergeld, Bernie, Ph.D. *The New Male Sexuality: The Truth About Men, Sex and Pleasure*. New York: Bantam Books, 1999.

Index by Director

Index by Film Title

ABOUT THE AUTHOR

VIOLET BLUE is senior copywriter at Good Vibrations, where she writes book and video reviews, which has her watching an awful lot of porn, and reading virtually everything imaginable about sex. She is a sex columnist and a sex educator. She is the editor of *Sweet Life: Erotic Fantasies for Couples* and *Sweet Life 2: Erotic Fantasies for Couples*, and the author of *The Ultimate Guide to Fellatio*, and *The Ultimate Guide to Cunnilingus*. Visit her web site: tinynibbles.com.